D0952916

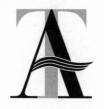

Books of Merit

Dangerous Lives

DANGEROUS LIVES

War and the Men and Women Who Report It

Anthony Feinstein

Thomas Allen Publishers
Toronto

National Library of Canada Cataloguing in Publication

Feinstein, A. (Anthony), 1956–
    Dangerous lives : war and the men and women who report it / Anthony Feinstein.

Includes index.

ISBN 0-88762-131-7

1. War correspondents—Mental health.   2. War correspondents—Psychology.
3. Psychic trauma.   I. Title.

PN4823.F43   2003   070.4'333'019   C2003-901999-3

Text design: Gordon Robertson
Editor: Janice Weaver
Jacket image: Christopher Morris/VII

"A Hazardous Profession: War, Journalists and Psychopathology" from the *American Journal of Psychiatry*, vol. 159, pp. 1550–575, September 2002, copyright 2002 the American Psychiatric Association; www.psychiatryonline.org. Reprinted by permission.

**Canada Council
for the Arts**

ONTARIO ARTS COUNCIL
CONSEIL DES ARTS DE L'ONTARIO

The publisher gratefully acknowledges the support of the Ontario Arts Council for its publishing program

We acknowledge the support of the Canada Council for the Arts, which last year invested $20.3 million in writing and publishing throughout Canada.

We acknowledge the Government of Ontario through the Ontario Media Development Corporation's Ontario Book Initiative.

07 06 05 04 03   1 2 3 4 5

Printed and bound in Canada

For John Owen

Happy the man who finds a generous friend.

— GREEK PROVERB

Contents

Introduction

I remember that night I sat bolt upright in bed.

I was living in Jerusalem as a correspondent for CBC Television. Earlier that day I had raced to the scene of a double suicide bombing. Within minutes of the explosions, Israeli soldiers and ambulances were everywhere. I was trying to get closer to the site of the actual blast when two men brushed by piloting an older woman through the chaos, towards a medic. She was able to walk, and had what appeared to be superficial cuts on her arms. She looked terrified. I found myself staring at her dark, shoulder-length hair, because the strands had clumped together unnaturally at the back. Why, in the midst of the carnage, would her hair even catch my attention? People had been killed. Palestinian bombers had targeted the main Jewish market and it was now a frightening tangle of mashed produce and mangled bodies. It would be a very long day of collecting very graphic and disturbing footage, and of writing it all out. I went home exhausted.

At some point in the small hours of the morning I awoke suddenly and startled myself by speaking aloud. "It was a wig." The woman was an ultra-Orthodox Jew. Her nylon wig had melted in the heat of the blast. I couldn't sleep; that single image bothered me too much. I had covered countless suicide bombings in Israel and witnessed wrenching scenes of human carnage. That night, the fused ends of a cheap wig became an unsettling symbol of the randomness of life and death in Jerusalem.

War for me comes back in sudden, unexpected ways. In a sound, a smell, an image. And then a memory wafts in, unstoppable and disturbing, if only for a moment. It is never about me, and it is rarely about the dead. It is about the pain of those who survive: a woman keening over the decomposed remains of her son. A child lying helpless in a hospital ward. A frontline soldier who sits down next to me to complain that this war has stolen his youth. I think of them still, and I wonder if I ever did them any justice, if anyone even cared about their stories when I tried to tell them. I wonder where they are today and ask myself why I haven't tried to find them again. Sometimes war comes back in denial, when an eager young journalist wants to hear my stories, and asks how many "close calls" I've had. I find those questions annoying, unwelcome. I know of too many journalists who have been killed or injured, so why talk of close calls?

A few years ago, sometime after I was in Bosnia and the Middle East, Anthony Feinstein contacted me and asked me to answer a long list of questions for a survey on Post-Traumatic Stress Disorder in war correspondents. I completed it carefully, from the safety of my office in Washington, D.C., the only survey I'd ever bothered to answer. I had been a foreign correspondent for CBC Television for about eight years at that point. I remember counting up my experiences covering wars, conflicts, a revolution, and one particularly devastating natural disaster, like so many notches in a belt, wondering if I'd covered enough death and destruction. Enough for what? I might have asked.

I have met or worked alongside many of the journalists in this book. As I read their stories, I can sometimes feel where they have been. I can feel the weight, the fatigue, even the adrenalin. I feel the guilt, too: the guilt of leaving, of not returning often enough, of not covering one war, of wondering if I really did make people back home understand the horror of people caught in conflict. Of course, these are not the emotions of the other reporters, they are mine. Feinstein has taken the information he's received from journalists and has sorted through their emotions, their pain, their relationships, and even their drinking habits to determine the toll that reporting on war takes on individuals. All the way through this book, many of them apologize for what they do. They all say, "We have tickets out," "We aren't the story," "I had to keep going back." Despite the best efforts of many to brush off their shattering experiences, Feinstein has found a thread, a common link in how work in dangerous places affects journalists.

Feinstein begins this book with the story of one perplexing patient, and as he works through her diagnosis, he introduces us to the work of journalists who cover war. Their experiences are beyond grisly, beyond what any human being would reasonably choose to witness. And yet we learn that most of them would be more disturbed if forced to stay away from conflict zones and their horrible realities. We meet the photographer whose breakdown comes after countless conflicts, snapping scenes of children blown to bits, of another crying blood. He breaks down in an airport, far from the terror his mind cannot escape. From Bosnia to Chechnya, from Rwanda to Sierra Leone to Lebanon, journalists accustomed to strife have unloaded their stories on Feinstein. A few admit to the adrenalin kick of putting their lives on the line to bring the news home; most insist their work is noble and necessary.

One journalist's story disturbed Feinstein so much that he flew to Uganda to learn more about him. We get a glimpse of the pressures on those who report on genocide and war in their own neighbourhoods. For them, there is no ticket home; they live in the region. The man Feinstein met in Uganda had covered countless African conflicts. After the massacre in Rwanda, he could no longer eat red meat. He adjusted his diet and kept on working because he really had no other choice. Feinstein attempted to help him, and in his story we learn how the simplest things become obstacles because of what they represent to someone who has witnessed far too much.

Remarkably, it is a minority of journalists who suffer serious effects of Post-Traumatic Stress Disorder. Feinstein discerns differences in men and women, in those who have partners and children, and those who do not. He chronicles variations in the behaviors of those faced with an immediate threat to their lives, from women taken captive, to those narrowly missed by mortars and bullets. He even looks at their drug and alcohol intake, and discovers a large number lead relatively well-adjusted lives despite their gruesome experiences and do not develop addictions. He examines those who finally get out and stay out, and those who are drawn back again and again. In the wake of the attacks on New York and Washington on September 11, 2001, he looks at domestic journalists dealing with the threat of terror and the pressure of news deadlines. Still, journalists who live and work in so much danger retain memories that many would not be able to fathom, and Feinstein forces them to talk about the images that linger, and the feelings that return.

For those he has interviewed, and those of us he has not, Feinstein has performed an important service to all journalists with this book. He has chronicled the effects of war on the people who chronicle the conflict; he has acknowledged and documented the pain such work exacts; he brings a new legitimacy to the concerns over reporters' long-term reactions to their work. As well, his work serves as a cautionary and instructive tool for the editors and news executives who make the decisions to send us to war. There are many journalists who are injured or killed in war. Feinstein reminds us that those who come home without physical injuries may still be bloodied psychologically, and their needs must not be ignored.

— Anna Maria Tremonti, June 2003

Dangerous Lives

1

A HAZARDOUS PROFESSION

Meanwhile, all across Rwanda, murder, murder, murder,
murder, murder, murder, murder, murder, murder . . .

— PHILIP GOUREVITCH

The patient who entered my office on a frigid December morning came with an interesting history. The referral note from the hospital's senior neurologist laid out the clinical details. The woman had suddenly taken ill in a restaurant while dining with family and friends. Her husband had noticed her ashen appearance and the beads of sweat on her brow and nose. When asked what the matter was, she had been unable to reply coherently. Alarmed by his wife's garbled speech, he had called for an ambulance.

En route to hospital, the woman lapsed in and out of consciousness, and by the time she arrived in the emergency room it was feared she had had a stroke. The neurology service was consulted and the patient sent for a brain CAT scan. To the surprise of the medical staff, no abnormality was seen, despite the persistence of her moribund state. She was admitted to hospital for further tests but by the following morning had made a spontaneous and complete recovery. At her own request she was discharged. She left the hospital smiling and seemingly in good spirits.

A week later, before she could keep her first outpatient appointment, the symptoms returned, suddenly and dramatically. One moment she was fine, calm and intelligible, the next, agitated, tremulous and incoherent. She was again rushed to hospital, where she was readmitted for more tests—scans that revealed the cerebral anatomy with postmortem-like clarity and showed how much blood was flowing to individual brain areas, electrodes that picked up the intensity and frequency of brain waves, multiple tubes of blood. All were normal. With methodical tenacity, the neurologist-in-chief worked his way through a long list of possible neurological causes for his patient's symptoms. Each was definitively ruled out. This done, he called in a cardiologist for an opinion. If there was nothing wrong with the brain, perhaps the problem lay with the heart and its ability to keep sufficient blood flowing to the brain. More tests followed. A mountain of computer printouts representing thousands of health-care dollars was distilled into a terse comment, scrawled in the patient's chart: "No abnormalities found." By this time, the patient had, as before, made a full recovery.

It was at this point that the woman was referred to my neuropsychiatric service. The typed letter from the neurologist-in-chief echoed Conan Doyle, whose lucid, deceptively simple prose and keen analytic mind he had long admired: "The physical examination is normal; the laboratory results are normal," he wrote. "When we have excluded the possible, whatever remains, however improbable, is the answer to the diagnostic riddle. I have therefore concluded there is nothing physically wrong with the patient." And then, almost as an afterthought, he had penned below his signature, in a beautiful flowing cursive, the following: "I wonder if it all has anything to do with her work? You may recognize the name. She's a war reporter."

It is not uncommon for patients to present with neurolo
symptoms that have no obvious physiological cause. Neurologists
will see many thousands of such patients a year. These patients are
said, in psychiatric parlance, to have a conversion disorder. This
is in effect a rerouting of emotional distress into physical symptoms, an unconscious process that changes, or converts, emotional
dysfunction into neurological abnormalities. The neurological
symptoms may be diverse, but they are invariably at odds with
the classic description of how they should behave. It is this
discrepancy that gives the clue to diagnosis. Patients with conversion disorder may be unable to speak, move limbs or experience
sensations such as touch and pain. What they all have in common,
despite the disparate set of complaints, is the absence of a neurological disorder that could account for their condition.

In the past these patients were given a diagnosis of hysteria.
The sometimes bizarre and florid nature of their symptoms would
seize the attention of the physician and even make for good theater.
The great nineteenth-century French behavioral neurologist Jean-
Martin Charcot routinely displayed such cases before a rapt audience at the Salpetrière Hospital in Paris. A famous painting by
Pierre André Brouillet, exhibited at the Salon de Paris in 1887,
shows Charcot and a swooning patient surrounded by an assort-
ment of onlookers—physicians, students, journalists, artists and
even Charcot's twenty-year-old son.

The often dramatic presentation of conversion disorder, coupled with the neurologist's sense that he may be missing some
underlying problem, frequently leads to a slew of unnecessary
investigations. Test after test is ordered, cementing within the
patients' minds a belief they are afflicted with serious physical
illness. And there is a compelling, albeit false, logic to that belief,
which is often unwittingly reinforced by the medical profession.
"Why do all the tests if you do not suspect something is seriously
wrong?" reasons the patient. If symptoms begin suddenly, if there

is a clearly identifiable stressor, and the patient is open to psychological explanations, the prognosis is often good.

In the case of the female journalist, the neurologist-in-chief had made the correct diagnosis. By the time she came to see me there was no trace of any language impediment, and the history I obtained was an articulate, compelling narrative of a work career spent in war zones. For years, I learned, this woman had led an itinerant life, following in the wake of armies and relief organizations and recording events that were for the most part brutal and desperately sad. A decade of cumulative stress, which had included a number of near-fatalities, reached an apogee when, in the span of a few days, her cameraman was killed while on assignment with her and, in a separate incident, a close colleague was badly wounded in an assassination attempt. Deeply shaken by these experiences, she had taken to medicating herself with tranquilizers and alcohol, two drugs that were readily available on the black market in war zones. She thought this would calm her nerves and give her a few hours of peaceful sleep, but instead her anxiety became acute; it was soon accompanied by a host of physical symptoms such as uncontrollable fits of shaking, sweating, a rapidly beating pulse and tightness in her chest. Frightened by these attacks, which she attributed to heart problems, she consulted a physician in Khartoum, who advised her to return to Canada for treatment. When she got back to her family in Toronto, however, some of her symptoms spontaneously disappeared. Buoyed by this improvement, she did not see a physician. It was a week after her return that she took ill in the restaurant.

It soon became clear in our conversations that while she loved her work as a war journalist, she found the job stressful and at times terrifying. The death of her cameraman and shooting of a close friend were not isolated events in a career that had seen colleagues killed and wounded at depressingly frequent intervals over the years. Still, although she counted many of those colleagues as friends, death had until recently bypassed her immediate circle and thus was viewed as something that happened to others but never to her. This charmed belief system suddenly disintegrated with the mortar shell that fell out of a clear blue African sky and took the life of her cameraman, someone with whom she had worked closely for five years.

As I gained more insights into her profession, I began to realize that the tragedy that had overtaken my patient was not unusual for a war reporter. So I was surprised when she told me that psychiatric help, even in the form of some basic counseling, was not readily available to her. Although she was employed by one of the world's major news organizations, she had no access to this type of assistance.

"There is an unspoken view within the profession that you either cut it or else get out," she told me. "There are no half measures. Reporting war is all about having the 'right stuff.' Sure, we know that we drink too much and at times our emotions are all screwed up, but that comes with the turf, and if you find that hard to deal with, then there is always the royal family to follow or a Wimbledon to report on, heaven forbid." She shuddered. She had by that time made the decision to give up working in conflict zones, but it was clear that domestic work had little appeal.

In the months since her first visit to the emergency room, I had persuaded her to cut back significantly on her alcohol consumption and begin exercising, and these two measures—coupled with medication to alleviate residual, at times intense, symptoms of anxiety—had brought about a considerable improvement in her mental state. She judged herself almost back to her old normal self, and her husband concurred.

Despite deciding not to return to front-line reporting, she remained haunted by her past and revisited these events in her therapy sessions with an obsessional regularity. The more I listened, the more I came to realize that her profession, for all its allure and excitement, was practiced at a cost to both emotional equilibrium and physical health. After a session in which she recalled, in moving terms, the famine in Sudan and how the images of that disaster refused to leave her, I turned to the medical literature to see what had been written about war journalists and their particular susceptibility to psychiatric distress. I imagined that a subject with such emotional impact would surely have stimulated a considerable body of work. No doubt I would be able to find some guidelines to long-term management and outcome, two variables that were of interest to me, given my patient's good early response to treatment.

A second surprise was in store. Not only had most of the news organizations neglected to provide for the psychological welfare of their war reporters, but trauma researchers had ignored them too. Trawling through the literature I could not find a single reference to the subject, no articles, chapters or abstracts. I had stumbled on a virgin topic, lying seemingly unrecognized within a larger literature devoted to the emotional consequences of traumatic events.

Matters could have been left, quite satisfactorily, at that. After all, the patient had recovered and I had learned from an interesting case. But the stories and images my patient had conveyed to me over the course of six months had more than piqued my curiosity. They had instilled within my researcher's mind a need to know more about this group of journalists, who, if my patient was any yardstick, chased wars, revolutions and famines with a tenacity both alarming and impressive. A host of questions had been stimulated by my contact with her. What kind of people chose war journalism as a career? What were the motivating factors that made them choose such a dangerous career? What were their backgrounds? What were their family lives like? Why had no one researched this area before? And central to the whole topic: how did war journalists react psychologically to the stresses and dangers of the job? In the case of my patient, the presentation had been florid, work-related stress masquerading as a constellation of neurological symptoms suggesting a stroke. Such a reaction struck me as extreme. But was it? I had no way of knowing. There were no data out there.

———

War journalists loom large in the public's consciousness. These intrepid men and women appear on prime-time television news against a backdrop of conflict and mayhem. The locations are frequently exotic, and the visual image is imbued with all the tension and drama that accompanies war. Any recent major conflict—Kosovo, Bosnia, the West Bank and Gaza, the Gulf War, Iraq—brings to mind images of flak-jacketed, helmeted reporters clutching microphones, while all around them smoke billows, buildings lie in ruins and explosions punctuate the dispatches. Their faces disappear and reappear as the media focus shifts from one part of the globe to another. But despite all the uncertainty and danger associated with war, their familiar presence remains one of the few constants. Somehow they appear untouched by the death and destruction that surrounds them and forms the heart of their métier.

This belief that war journalists are removed from the events they report on is captured perfectly by Jules Verne. His richly imagined novel *Mysterious Island* begins with the escape of four Union soldiers by balloon from a military prison in Richmond, Virginia, during the American Civil War. After surmounting many hazards the men find themselves marooned on an island, where their fight for survival is aided by Captain Nemo of the submarine *Nautilus*. On meeting the group for the first time, the mysterious captain tells one of the escapees, Gideon Spillet, a war correspondent with the *New York Herald*, "I know you. You specialize in war news. You supply the ink, the soldiers supply the blood." Spillet does not challenge the captain's opinion, and his silence may be construed as tacit agreement that this is indeed how his profession operates. Soldiers may bleed and die, but journalists emerge unscathed. And is this not how it should be? After all, war journalists are not combatants, the conflict is not theirs and they do not bear arms. They simply have a job to do, which is to report the news, and night after night their presence in millions of homes is testimony to Nemo's trenchant opinion.

Jules Verne was not alone in his view. Over the past twenty years a burgeoning literature has focused on how individuals deal with potentially life-threatening stressors. A formidable psychological trauma industry has been spawned, with few traumas left unexplored. Researchers have examined how veterans respond to the dangers of combat and civilians cope with man-made and natural disasters. Rape victims, assault victims, refugees, policemen, firemen, abused spouses and children, survivors of motor vehicle and industrial accidents—all have been studied in depth and their psychological responses to trauma documented. Yet, as I discovered, nowhere in the countless pages devoted to psychological trauma is there a single piece of research on war journalists.

To a degree, the profession itself has helped foster this silence. Entrenched within the persona of the war journalist is an element of self-deception—the idea that he or she is someone who can confront war with impunity. It could be argued that this is a prerequisite. The news bosses are not immune to this way of thinking either, for it affords them a degree of comfort when dispatching journalists to wherever the latest conflagration erupts. So effective has the profession been in fortifying these constructs and perpetuating a very public myth of unassailability that researchers in the field of psychological stress have, to date, passed them by.

But cracks have started to appear in the well-constructed defenses. Organizations such as Reporters Sans Frontières and the Canadian-based International Freedom of Expression Exchange (IFEX) now keep statistics on the number of journalists arrested, tortured, wounded and killed. Their communiqué for the year 2000 lists sixty-two journalists who were assassinated. While the majority of these were local reporters killed for exposing crime

and corruption, the names of war journalists also figure prominently. The deaths in Sierra Leone of two celebrated and very
experienced journalists, Kurt Schork of Reuters and Miguel Gil
Moreno of Associated Press Television News, have helped challenge the notion of invulnerability that has so tightly enveloped the
profession.

———

Chris Cramer is just one journalist who has suffered work-related
psychological trauma. What makes him different is not that he displayed such unusual symptoms, but that he has written with candor
about his experience. In 1980, when he was a field producer with
the British Broadcasting Corporation, Cramer went to the Iran-
ian embassy in London to apply for a visa. He wanted to go to
Tehran to report on the American hostage drama that was then
unfolding. He had been standing in a lineup for only a few minutes
when six terrorists stormed the embassy and took him and others
hostage. Held for thirty-six hours, he escaped by faking a heart
attack. The remaining hostages were freed by his country's Special
Air Services (SAS) six days later. After the siege had ended,
Cramer was offered stress counseling by the BBC and the Home
Office. He rejected both, a decision he later came to regret. "It
wasn't the done thing, but I think if I knew then what I know now, I
would have taken myself off to a shrink."

Like many who have been exposed to hazardous situations,
Cramer found that the event lived on in his mind in the weeks,
months and years ahead, not only influencing his emotions and
behavior but also acting at times as the catalyst for life-changing
decisions. "It fundamentally changed my ability to do my job," he
recalled. "In other words, I lost my bottle. I did not want to be
knowingly anywhere that was unsafe—at one point, that could
even be a restaurant or the underground. I didn't want to be
anywhere that put things outside my control." Six months after

the siege he moved from reporting the news into a management position at the BBC.

Today Cramer is president of CNN International Networks. Sensitized by his own experience, he has used his present position to facilitate a debate on what can be done to help war journalists traumatized by their work. He is not alone in his concern. The BBC established a policy of offering counseling to employees back in the 1990s, and other news organizations are starting to follow suit. An overall concern for journalists' physical safety seems to have led to a newfound willingness on the part of the news organizations to discuss their psychological safety as well. This told me it was a good time to initiate the first organized study of the effects of stress and trauma on war journalists.* However, before I could even begin to assess the extent of the problem—if indeed there was one—I needed to develop an understanding of what war journalists experience in bringing the news to the public at large. Many in the profession are skilled wordsmiths, and their accounts of what they have endured are frequently articulate and imbued with all the passion of the events witnessed. Accordingly, letting them speak in their own words has certain important advantages—better to hear this direct than have it filtered through the word processor of the researcher.

---

* I was initially uncertain what to call the study's participants. The terms "foreign correspondents" or "war correspondents," while widely used, would not capture the stills photographers, television cameramen/women and producers covering conflict. For similar reasons, the label "war reporters" was considered too limiting. In the end, I opted for "war journalists," but I recognize that people such as the BBC's John Simpson dislike the term. In his memoirs, he describes an episode in which, in the presence of Martha Gellhorn, he berated his colleague Max Hastings for using the words. Simpson's objection is that some journalists may use the "war" descriptor as a means to self-aggrandizement. While in certain cases he may be correct, none of the journalists in my study did so. It is also important to point out that the journalists I studied did not confine their work to war zones. War and conflict, however, formed such a large and defining part of their careers that the term seems appropriate.

Anthony Loyd is a journalist working for the London *Times*. The author of a painfully candid memoir, *My War Gone By: I Miss It So*, he has reported in Bosnia, Croatia, Albania, Kosovo, Afghanistan, Nigeria, Ethiopia and Syria. But the conflict that stands out for him as the most dangerous was Chechnya.

"Chechnya was the most shocking because the violence was so intense and the war so encompassing," he told me. "There was a guarantee that if you scrambled out of your basement and went out into the city center, you either saw people getting killed or people who had just been killed or were terribly wounded. Or you would have a near death experience yourself."

Loyd arrived in Chechnya in the winter of 1994 and stayed for six weeks. The level of violence in Russia's breakaway republic was so extreme that many journalists had opted to stay away. In besieged Grozny, he found a city under such intense bombardment that there was no place for journalists to hunker down and wait out the danger. "I can generally expose myself to violence for a period of time if I want to and then go back to some safe place at the end of the day," Loyd explained. "Once you were in Grozny, however, there was none of that, and the image I have taken away is one of the sudden explosion of shells and then people sprayed all over the walls. . . .

"One experience particularly sticks with me. There was a heavy barrage going on outside the basement I was holed up in with four or five colleagues, and then it stopped and this young Russian girl came rushing in and was shouting in her broken English, 'Help us, help us.' We ran off with her into the snow, and not very far away we ran smack into this woman, a big woman covered in blood and wearing a fur coat—I don't know if it was her blood—and she was dragging a sledge and on the sledge was, I don't know who, her husband or brother or whatever. He was dead, in bloody shreds, a twisted torso—with one leg dragging off it. They must have been walking along with something else on the sledge, and then he must have been killed by the shelling and she probably just rolled him onto the sledge. In her hand she had his other leg—a big leg—with the boot on. She was completely unhinged by what had happened maybe half a minute before, and she was screaming at us, as close as I am to you, with this leg going back and forth, this big fucking leg—and you could just see in the gap between her gloves and coat, her skin, taut with the effort from the weight of the leg, and she was screaming at us. We were transfixed, and lying just behind her, where this barrage of shells had landed, were about six or seven people—her own people, actually—who had been just blown to bits lying around with bits of head and limb and everything."

Groznaya. The word in Russian means "terrible." And terrible indeed were the sights that Loyd confronted. Amid the carnage an old man lay facedown, covered in dust. Both legs had been severed, one above the knee, the other below. As Loyd walked past the stricken man a hand reached out and grabbed his ankle. "He was still alive! The heat of the blast had actually cauterized his wounds. He was not even bleeding. I was just in shock," recalled Loyd. "What the fuck to do? I mean, you are in this place where there is no hospital and there is no car, there is heavy fighting everywhere, there were no people on the streets because of the fighting and even the fighters are inside taking shelter and then you confront this horrible mutilation and this one old guy is still alive without his legs! We could hear the raining barrage of shells that were sort of fixed in lines to fire and going off all over the place. Possibly there were thirty shells suddenly exploding and maybe coming closer to us ... or maybe not—it was impossible to gauge.

"There was this really heavy fear between me and these other three guys, and we just looked at each other, and this old man could tell what was happening. I can speak a bit of Russian and could understand what he was saying. He kept grabbing my legs, saying, 'My legs, my legs. Please don't leave me, please don't leave me,' and we ran because we were fucking frightened. I think we were really shell-shocked—and mutilation is really distressing to witness—so we ran back to our cellar. A couple of the other journalists were trying to say that the Russian girl had come because she wanted us to film what had happened because she felt that it was bad and wanted journalists to show the world. I am fucking sure that she did not come for that reason. I'm sure she came because she wanted us to help."

For Anthony Loyd, six years on, the memories of that terrible scene in Grozny remain vivid. He had seen many people killed in conflict before, but that day, and particularly the image of the woman waving the leg, is engraved on his memory. "It's like looking at a light bulb and then looking at the afterimage. Days later, I could still see that woman. Literally for several days after it, there was this serum of an imprint. I still think of the image very often. I certainly have not forgotten it."

One of the other journalists who was in Grozny on that fateful winter's day was the freelancer Jon Jones. A veteran of photographing conflict over a fifteen-year period, Jones too regarded Grozny as his most dangerous assignment, but for him it's not the actual fighting or even his own close calls that disturb him the most. Rather, what moves Jones is the fallout of the fighting—that is, the effects of war on the local population and the destruction it brings to their lives.

On one occasion Jones and some other journalists were taken to a hospital to view the victims of a Russian bombing attack on a Chechen farm. There he met two sisters; the older one, who was about nine, was badly wounded, but it was the younger one, about eight, who really affected him. "She was unscathed," he remembers, "covered in mud, but she was crying blood. She had blood running down her cheeks from the concussion effects of the bombs. After that visit, we were taken to the farm [where the bombing had occurred], and it had been devastated. They took us into this little room, and there was this bed just full of dismembered children. There were about eight or nine of them under these blankets. They were in pieces, literally in pieces. You can't shoot it. You can't. What I used to do was shoot a frame or two in acknowledgment that I had been there and had seen it and as a way of showing my editors I had been there. But I knew it wasn't going to go anywhere. Nobody is going to publish it. So you do it because you are there to record it, but you don't make a thing of it. . . . The picture I have is of a child's head and just a blanket, but they took the blanket off, and it's like, 'You can't do that, put the blanket back on.' That and the image of the girl crying blood stay with me."

———————

Why repeat stories like these? What is to be achieved by describing the minutiae of a massacre? Is it not sufficient to state that war journalists are exposed to danger and see gruesome sights? After all, a degree of self-imposed media censorship is already taking place, as alluded to by Jon Jones. Even as he focused his lens on the bed of dismembered children, he knew the few frames he shot were going nowhere. The images were simply unprintable, the horror of the episode deemed beyond what the public could stomach. However, when news organizations sanitize the content of news, pandering to their viewers' sensitivities, they also inadvertently influence the public's perception of just how dangerous war journalism is.

This point is pivotal on many levels because it is the experience of war that defines the profession and the very essence of those who practice it. This is also what drives the symptoms that live on long after the events and captures the public's imagination so vividly. However, maintaining a balance between factual description on the one hand and sensationalism on the other demands vigilance. Fascination with what the war journalist endures in war zones can very easily slip into voyeurism. This does the profession and any study of it a disservice. Conversely, to back off from describing the full magnitude and breadth of the dangers confronted by war journalists would leave the impression that it was indeed ink that was more likely to be spilled. Extending an anodyne to the lives of war journalists would also make any meaningful psychological study of the profession impossible. For the reader to discern the significance of war journalists' dreams or flashbacks, to comprehend the strains placed on their relationships and the difficulties many have in adjusting to life back in a society not racked by conflict, then war, and the pity of war, in Wilfred Owen's memorable words, must be laid bare. It is a theme that will reappear throughout this book; if readers are to understand what war journalists do, the sanitized wrapping placed around war must be stripped away.

The lives of war journalists are, to varying degrees, bound to the lives of the perpetrators and, more commonly, the victims of war. And being war's amanuensis can come at a cost. In Bosnia in 1989, Jon Jones experienced firsthand the terror of being cast as a target by Serbian paramilitary forces. "On a number of occasions I was taken into the wood at midnight and had a mock execution. Twice I was dragged out of a car and put up against a wall. I thought that was it. They stripped me of all identification. You can tell that you are in trouble when you hand over your passport and a guy spits on it and throws it into the bushes. They thought we were spies. They were hassling us, intimidating us, trying to force us into speaking Serbian or Croatian, which someone would do the more scared he got [when people tend to revert to their mother tongue]. Finally it was clear we couldn't speak either language, so they let us go, and I remember climbing into the car and I was shaking. I couldn't drive. It was a real effort.

"It happened in Grozny as well. Pro-Russian rebels took me into a wood in a car, and I tried to get out and they kicked the door shut. I thought, This is it. They'll just waste me in the car. They didn't. I was there for about an hour. They made me drive to the front line at two o'clock in the morning, which is even more dangerous. Luckily I was fine. Those kinds of things would just happen."

There is not just the element of brinkmanship on the part of these rogue militia. At times, threats translate into action. The case of Fred Cluny is a tragic example of this. William Shawcross, in his book *Deliver Us from Evil*, has called Cluny a "great American—a sort of universal Schindler, a man with lists of millions of people . . . whose lives he succoured and saved." Cluny coupled his technical expertise in urban planning with a remarkable gift for improvisation and force of character to spearhead humanitarian relief operations, first in Biafra and thereafter wherever conflict or disaster demanded the attention of the world's non-governmental organizations—Bangladesh, Cambodia, Guatemala, Armenia, the Gulf War, Kuwait, Somalia, Bosnia, Albania and finally Chechnya, where he went missing with two Russian Red Cross doctors and a woman interpreter. Despite the efforts of many, from President Clinton down, he was never found until years later, when some Chechens claiming to have his body offered it as ransom to his family. Such is the randomness of war. On a whim, the callous, and to us inexplicable, impulse of a bandit warlord or one of his minions—a life embracing a quarter century of the most remarkable humanitarianism is snuffed out.

Sitting captive in his car in the Chechen woods, Jon Jones knew that those who kill so easily seldom weigh their actions on the scales of justice. "Where there is anarchy you can do anything you want," he said in an interview with me. "That's why soldiers just go berserk. If soldiers take a town they don't stop killing. Once all the defenders have gone they kill everything—birds, dogs, cows, chickens. They don't stop until it's all gone."

We paused in the interview and Jones lit a cigarette. Having listened to him relate several other harrowing escapes I asked an obvious question: Have experiences like these ever made him think of doing something else for a living? In response, he got up from the kitchen table and walked over to a noticeboard, removed a pin and handed me a photograph that shows a room with a hole in the wall, the faint pattern of wallpaper, smashed furniture at the head of a bed.

"The only time I thought of that was when I had a shell in my bed," he told me quietly. "I was lying in bed at night—this is Sarajevo—and a mortar tank from the local army pulled up outside my front door and started firing at the Serbs. This is a regular thing they do. But normally they fire four or five rounds and then run. This time it was eight, nine, ten, eleven rounds. The first round of returning fire hits the building next to me . . . and the second round came through my wall. It was an artillery round, and it came through the wall into a chest of drawers that my bed was up against and exploded and blew me right across the room into another wall. And I hadn't got a mark on me, not a scratch. But I was wet. I started panicking because I thought it was blood. A friend of mine ran in from the next room with a torch. It was milk. A big carton of milk had exploded. So I was covered in milk, covered in plaster dust, just standing there."

———

I came to observe that the violence inflicted on war journalists, either by accident or intent, was at times indistinguishable from that endured by the civilian population in the areas of conflict. What befell the photographer John Liebenberg on the battlefields of northern Namibia and Angola in the late 1980s and 1990s illustrates both the randomness and premeditated nature of this threat. Liebenberg was on the staff of the *Namibian*, a newspaper that was a vocal and barely tolerated opponent of South African occupation. His photographs of atrocities committed against SWAPO (South West African People's Organization) fighters by members of Koevoet, a lawless Namibian police group closely allied to South Africa, led to his frequent arrest and maltreatment. On one occasion he was incarcerated in a room with a wild baboon. "The animal was really savage," he recalled. "It had bitten people and sat there snarling at me. . . . And that fear . . . that sweat . . . is still with me."

Despite such intimidation, he persisted in his work, even after a bounty was placed on his head. When independence finally came to Namibia, Liebenberg turned his attention to the civil war in neighboring Angola. His personal archive of horror accumulated in Portugal's erstwhile colonial jewel is of a magnitude that is extraordinary and unsettling to record. "I was very fortunate to have known some of the generals in Luanda who gave me access to the front lines. One day I flew into an area recently captured from UNITA (National Union for the Total Independence of Angola), and the MPLA (Popular Movement for the Liberation of Angola) general gave an order that looters would be shot. That afternoon two boys were brought to him. They had been caught raping some women. They were angry that UNITA people had been living in their house. The general just took out his pistol and shot one of the youngsters in the groin and the other in the stomach and then he sat back in his chair. The boys were in agony, asking for water, crying, oh my god and the commander looked over at me and said, 'If you give these guys water, my friend, I will fucking kill you now.'" A shocked Liebenberg ignored the threat. He was fortunate. The general did not shoot him too. His penalty was to be placed back in the helicopter and banished from the front lines for a week. But the episode, like many others, stayed with him. "Instead of trying to describe how I feel about it today, let me just say I don't photograph weddings and I won't photograph baptisms because I cry," he confided.

In Liebenberg's tortured Angolan narrative, there is a hurried sense of inevitability about future calamity. "In 1997, the plane I was traveling in crashed near Huambo, one of the districts in central Angola. . . . We were coming in to land, in a tight spiral. UNITA had just left the fringes of the city, but elements had stayed behind, and a group fired a missile at the plane. It hit a wing, [and] the plane crashed. . . . The pilots were killed, and some of my colleagues were really badly injured. . . . After the crash, the plane exploded. . . . It was quite close to a battalion of young MPLA soldiers, tank soldiers, and they immediately started looting the plane . . . and there I was with a serious bang on the head, trying to get my equipment and stuff out."

The experiences of Anthony Loyd, Jon Jones and John Liebenberg are not unusual. They are repeated time and again by others, with a relentless intensity over the course of many years. Greg Marinovich, Joao Silva, Ken Oosterbroek and Kevin Carter were four South African photographers who traveled the unpaved streets and alleys of the sprawling black ghettoes of Johannesburg to produce a series of shocking images, documenting their country's transition from shamefaced polecat to regional powerhouse. The time of greatest danger is when a bad regime starts to reform, observed Alexis de Tocqueville. South Africa in the early 1990s was the perfect affirmation of this. Rampaging mobs, murder by stabbing, necklacing, the panic of crowds fired on by the security police, the summary roadside execution of white supremacists by a black soldier—their pictures gained them national and international prominence and awards followed, including a Pulitzer Prize for Marinovich for an image of a man stabbed and set alight by a crazed mob. The four photographers quickly became known as the Bang-Bang Club, and in turn the subject of articles and photographs that recorded their hazardous lives. By the time South Africa limped into its first multiracial general election, the toll exerted by the unremitting violence on the Bang Bang Club was appalling. Oosterbroek had been killed, Carter had committed suicide, and Marinovich had been shot. Only Silva emerged physically unscathed. Adding to the attrition, an unofficial fifth member of the group, the photographer Gary Bernard, also committed suicide. The two surviving members have told their story in a book that became the vehicle for a cathartic outpouring of pent-up grief and anger.

Marinovich's career is an example of the risks war journalists encounter. He has been wounded four different times, once during the confrontation that claimed the life of Oosterbroek. On that fateful day, the members of the Bang Bang Club had gone to Thakosa to photograph a looming showdown between rival militias. Members of the National Peacekeeping Force (NPKF), a conglomeration of troops from the South African police, apartheid homeland armies and the South African Defence Force were meant to storm a hostel occupied by Inkatha fighters. But the poorly trained peacekeepers panicked, firing their weapons indiscriminately, killing Oosterbroek and seriously wounding Marinovich.

It is a day Marinovich will never forget, but his initial reaction was not what we might expect. "The most interesting sensation was, after the pain and the shock of those first few minutes, that when I thought I was going to die, there was this massive relief. Because of all the feelings I was telling you about—this guilt, this voyeurism, this profiting through the whole thing, always escaping unhurt, having covered various conflicts by then and with varying degrees of caring about what I was doing. So there was this relief of having finally paid my dues, making up for what I've photographed. Being scared was no longer there, it wasn't there."

Marinovich was rushed to hospital, where his condition deteriorated and fear returned, intermingled with grief for his dead friend, who was lying nearby. "My pulse was dropping, and I couldn't breathe properly because my lung had collapsed. Some friends came into the hospital ER with TV cameras and instead of rolling, they were just looking at me. Very experienced people and I thought, Fuck, I'm going to die."

Marinovich is a large, pleasantly disheveled man with an open, forthright manner. His answers come quickly, emotionally. There is a no-nonsense warmth to him. Like those of many of the journalists I have interviewed, his descriptions of events are often scatological. Marinovich likes the word *fuck*. Fuck this, fuck that, racist fucks. We chatted on the rooftop of a Johannesburg hotel. After the trauma of the past decade, the period when we spoke was an exciting, happy time for him and Joao Silva. Their photographic skills had received international acclaim, their book, *The Bang-Bang Club*, was about to be launched, and there was talk of a movie. His cell phone rang constantly. After speaking to his fiancée who had phoned from Switzerland, he turned the phone off and we resumed talking.

Three months after he was shot, financial pressures pushed him into an ill-timed assignment, and he developed a series of lung infections and gout, all complications of his initial surgery. In the end he needed almost a year to recover fully. Another shooting followed five months after the first—"the police opened up with birdshot and I was wounded all over; not traumatic"—and a third three years after that. This one, during the South African invasion of Lesotho, was more serious.

"That was terrifying. Joao [Silva] plus myself and Suzanne [Daley, the chief correspondent from the *New York Times*] got caught in ambush after ambush with South African soldiers. We got Suzanne into a safe spot, and we went up to the armored vehicles that were pinned down under ambush. We were doing very good pictures. There were bullets around and it was quite scary, but there was this excitement because they were soldiers, not civilians. There's a difference, you know what I mean? Then we got out of that situation and parked the car quite a distance away and decided not to take further chances, just wait for the South Africans to finish mopping up and then go in. And a machine gun opened up on us where we were parked. I started the car, drove off and stalled, or the anti-hijack device kicked in. And we just kept taking this machine-gun fire. As I stalled I got hit in the leg . . . but I didn't say anything as I had to keep the car going. We drove another kilometer under constant fire, completely terrified, and that magic bubble had disappeared yet again, that bubble of invincibility. 'Cause until you're hit, you're immortal, right? That's what happened in the first shooting. Once you're hit, you feel very vulnerable to this kind of stuff. That magic bubble is gone."

Listening to Greg Marinovich I discerned a common thread linking his thinking to that of Loyd, Jones, Liebenberg and almost all the other war journalists who spoke to me of their experiences. They operate within a unique belief system, one that defines the concepts of threat and danger quite differently from any other group of subjects I have studied. It is not that their appreciation of what constitutes danger is absent, but rather that the threshold of what, for them, defines risk has been shifted so far along the continuum of our shared beliefs as to make it difficult to detect. How else to interpret what Joao Silva had to tell me. "I've been injured. Twice in fact. But all minor details. I've never been shot. I was injured in a grenade explosion and took a bit of shrapnel in my lower elbow. The second incident was during a riot. I got smashed in the face with a brick. It took me out of commission for a couple of days. I've never been injured in the sense that I've been hospitalized for months, so it doesn't really count." Or the immediate reaction of Jon Jones to the mortar shell that smashed through his wall: "I was furious, really kind of angry about the whole thing, you know. Saturday night. Midnight. I don't mind it during the day when I'm looking for it."

———

Fergal Keane was one of forty war journalists whose names were given to me by the BBC. My first contacts with him had been via e-mail, and in those brief exchanges, as we passed messages back and forth trying to set up a date and time for an interview, I became aware of this articulate, eager voice, impatient to share his thoughts on why journalists choose war as their subject and the consequences of that choice on their psyches. We finally met in his west London home on a blustery, wet and cold winter's morning. My first impressions of the man, gleaned from e-mail correspondence, were confirmed. He brings an intensity and energy to the discussion that demands attention. We spoke of many topics pertaining to war journalists, including the physical dangers they confront;

their relationships with family, friends and news bosses; the question of whether the profession is becoming more dangerous over time; the difficulty of maintaining journalistic neutrality in a conflict; and the problem of substance abuse within the profession. For the most part the conversation flowed easily, but whenever it derailed, the reason inevitably was Rwanda.

Keane had already covered several African conflicts, including the war between Ethiopia and Eritrea and the run-up to the first multiracial general election in South Africa, by the time he went to Rwanda in 1994. But nothing could have prepared him for the genocide he encountered there. It was clear to me, almost eight years later, that his Rwandan experiences had left an indelible impression. Even for Fergal Keane, the most articulate of men, the horror was on a scale that made it ineffable.

"We lived out in the field. There was no hotel to go back to at the end of the day. So, we lived with the victims in abandoned villages, with the smell of the corpses around. And I suppose I found it incredibly frightening because half the journey [from the border to the town of Butari] was through areas controlled by the genocidal forces, the Interahamwe [the Hutu militia], and that was the kind of fear I'd never experienced before. . . . It was more than just personally dangerous. The tensions were frightening, but this was a level beyond. There was a degree to which the whole moral order was gone, so killing was the right thing to do. There were no boundaries and everyone around had this kind of blood frenzy. . . . We felt very threatened. There were maybe thirty roadblocks between the Burundi border and Butari, and negotiating them was just petrifying. The Interahamwe would come up and hold grenades in the window, by the pin, and you were trying to persuade them you weren't Belgian because they wanted to kill any Belgians. That was terrifying."

Keane's first Rwandan visit lasted three weeks. He has come to look back on it as the most difficult and frightening period of his

career. When he returned to the country soon after the slaughter
had abated, the emotional residue of that first experience clung
tenaciously.

"When I was first in the country we saw a group of Tutsis,
survivors who had not been killed, outside the mayor's office. We
went and we filmed, and then we went back again that night to try
to film them again, but we were turned away at gunpoint. We were
told by a priest that these people had been taken and killed that
night, and we were too scared to go back and do anything about it.
I felt a lot of guilt about that.

"On the last day of my second trip, we met a woman who had
been in Butari at the time, a Tutsi survivor. She turned out to be one
of those people who were in front of the mayor's office, and she said
that she remembered us coming. She then said something that
was really devastating. She said, 'We thought you were with the
militia because you did nothing to help us. We thought you must
be with them.' And she said that three busloads of them were taken
away, and the militia killed two busloads and then they ran out of
energy for killing. I said to her, 'Look, I want you to know I'm sorry,
but I was too afraid at the time.' We were too afraid to do anything.
I mean, it's hard to convey to you the level of fear in a situation
like that."

I had completed twenty-six interviews with war journalists
by the time I came to interview Keane. For the most part the
interviews took place in their homes or in local cafés. There had
been no prior contact between me and my subjects other than
an exchange of letters, faxes or e-mails. To begin my study, I first
collected detailed questionnaires from 140 war journalists (out
of 170 names) given to me by respected news organizations,
including CNN, the BBC, Reuters, the Associated Press Television
News, NBC, ITN, the CBC and the Rory Peck Trust (an organization of freelance camerapeople, named after one of the most
respected freelancers of his generation, a man killed in crossfire
while covering the October coup and demonstrations outside

Moscow's television center in 1993). The thirty journalists who did not respond either could not be traced or politely refused, save one. "I happen to be just amazed about the questionnaire I found in my mail," he wrote. "The first sheet happened to ask me how many cans of beer I could drink in a week and if I was a cocaine addict.* You might know we are a very small community of war correspondents, and my friends might have the same feeling: are we all supposed to be neurotic, alcoholic, overstressed depressed jerks, permanently flirting with suicidal ideas? Should I rush to a psychoanalyst's couch if I consider myself—and am widely considered—a well-balanced father of two, normally stressed in a stressful profession, enjoying parties like any average thirty-six-year-old human being? Anyway, I am retired from the job now, being a correspondent in Washington. So you won't be offended if I don't answer your questionnaire. At least it did have a positive impact on my depression: a huge laugh. Respectfully yours . . ."

———

The second phase of my study involved face-to-face interviews with a random sample of one in five war journalists. These twenty-eight interviews took place in London, New York, Paris, Madrid, Barcelona and Johannesburg, and together with the information from the questionnaires, they form the basis of this book. To control for the stressors generic to journalism, such as getting the scoop and pressured deadlines, a group of 107 domestic journalists who had never been to war or disaster zones underwent the same assessment procedure (questionnaires and interviews for one in five). When I discuss the findings, reference will be made to this group as well.

The journalists who took part in my study were largely male (more than 70 percent) and mostly in their late thirties or early

---

* In fact, the questionnaire did neither of these things.

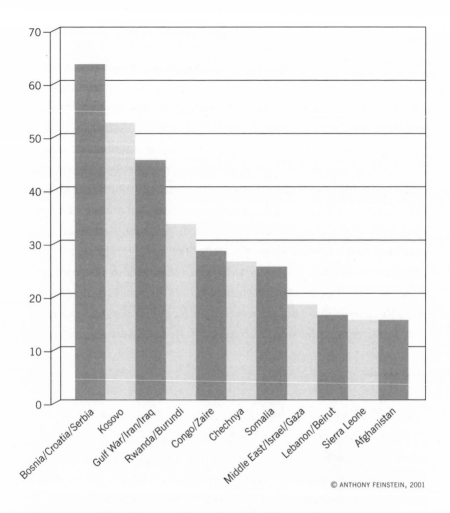

© ANTHONY FEINSTEIN, 2001

Percentage of War Correspondents Covering Various Locations

forties. The war group were also experienced, having spent on average fifteen years covering wars. Among them, they had written about or filmed every late-twentieth-century conflagration, big and small. More than 70 percent had been to the Balkans, making this region the most widely covered of the many conflict zones listed. (Contrast this with the 33 percent who went to Rwanda, the less than 20 percent who had covered Sierra Leone, or the single photojournalist who found his way to Angola, the locale of Africa's

longest-running war. Clearly, reporting Africa was not a top priority for organizations and their journalists.) Other trouble spots
visited by the journalists included Lebanon during the civil war
of the early 1980s, the Gulf War of the early 1990s, Chechnya,
Ngorno-Karabakh, East Timor, Israel, Gaza and the West Bank,
Afghanistan, the Congo, Ethiopia, Eritrea, Sudan, South Africa,
Namibia and El Salvador.

All the war journalists contacted for interviews were willing
to speak with me. After a decade or more in combat zones there
was much to tell, but every journalist had, in his repository of
hundreds of traumatic memories, a particular event that stood out
with an eidetic quality. Most of these fell into one of two categories.
The first, applicable to the majority, involved narrowly escaping
death—getting wounded, or being shot at, or having their plane
shot down—as detailed earlier in this chapter. What intrigued me
was the second type of response. Here the event, and for the most
part it was seldom more than a single event, did not necessarily
involve anything life-threatening. Nor did it involve witnessing
scenes of mutilation or wide-scale destruction. Rather, it centered
on the survivors of war, the victims who through some peculiar
twist in fate had been spared death only to confront their own shattered existence. It was the plight of the distraught—people who
had lost their children, families, livelihood, homes and communities; people who were overtaken by events often not of their making and devastated by the magnitude of their loss—that shocked
the journalists' sensibilities, outraged their morality or triggered
compassion and pity. And it was one or any combination of these
reactions that coalesced around the image and seared it into their
consciousness.

Thus, for some of these men and women who had witnessed
death and dying of almost biblical proportions, it was not death
itself but rather the consequences of death that provided the most
memorable and troubling recollections. "At times I felt like an
undertaker, seeing the number of bodies," Jeremy Bowen, the

BBC's Middle East Correspondent told me. "After having seen [a body] for the first time in El Salvador . . . going from that to the ridiculous, with piles of corpses, terribly mangled. I remember an event, the missile attack on the Amiriya shelter in Baghdad during the Gulf War, the so-called command bunker. . . . We got to the site a couple of hours after it happened. They were pulling out the most horrendous bits of bodies—not just bodies, but bits of bodies—and later we went to the morgue where they had taken them. . . . You walked into the building, the corridors were full of bodies. There was a big pathology lecture theater, with two slabs at the bottom and tiered seating, like in a university. The slabs had bodies on them, the floors and the tiered seating of the lecture theater had bodies on them. We were literally walking around like this [and here Jeremy Bowen rose on his toes to demonstrate the absence of floor space], picking our way around the things. So going from not seeing bodies at all to that place and watching the cameraman trying to put his tripod up, trying to find place on the floor for his tripod, and between the legs of the tripod was a corpse. A lot of them were terribly mangled, but what was worse was the grief of the survivors. I always find that is the case. Death is nasty, but it ends there for the dead."

When sympathy for the survivors merges into personal identification with them, the resultant image assumes a different emotional valence, making it deeply moving, disturbing and thus unforgettable. It often takes very little to bring this about. "Dead is dead. It's all the same, really," confided Jon Jones. "Sometimes the worst things aren't the carnage. The worst things are people you can relate to, people who look like your mother or sister."

Having to varying degrees become habituated to death and the misery of whole populations displaced, journalists may find that suddenly confronting something familiar in one of the bereaved or dispossessed—and it may be no more than the shape of a mouth or nose, a particular tilt to the head or some subtle, idiosyncratic mannerism—is enough to shatter the cocoon of detachment and force the tragedy of some nameless victim into that well-defended, inviolable frame of personal reference. With the wall breached, an array of fears and anxieties previously held at bay by fortified psychological defenses may be let in, further magnifying the emotional impact of the image. This, then, is the memory that some war journalists select, with little hesitation, from a decade-long catalog of traumatic experiences, and the speed with which they make their choice, coupled with the clarity of their recall, highlights the power of the personalized image to capture the imagination.

There is also a third type of experience, one that I have touched on only briefly thus far. It concerns loss, the death of a colleague who may have been a close friend too. It is the most emotive of topics and it has affected every war journalist I interviewed. No one has escaped it, everyone is conscious of it and the threat posed by it hovers over them all, introducing an additional tension to the work they do. For this is a small, tightly knit group of men and women, and the death of one is felt collectively. The loss of colleagues, introducing as it does guilt and self-reappraisal, is a theme central to the profession, one linked inextricably to the nature of the war journalist's experience.

In time I also came to realize that the experience helps explain who journalists are as people. In my correspondence and in the many hours of taped interviews, the drama of lives devoted to recording war, with all its excitement and wonder, tragedy and pathos, were laid bare. It's a heady concoction, and an unknown source sums it up well. "You may call war damnable—there is nothing too bad that can be said about it—and yet, it has a knack, which peace never learned, of uncovering the splendor in commonplace persons."

That insight is applicable, in varying measures, to both war's combatants and its victims. It holds true also for war journalists— their anecdotes are testimony to the extraordinary lengths they go to in order to document the news. Therein lies their paradox: war as the catalyst, not nemesis, to their creativity. In this chapter I have relayed but a few of the many experiences conveyed to me. For the men and women of my study have led not only dangerous lives, they have been busy too, in a decade that, according to the International Red Cross, saw over fifty-six wars, resulting in seventeen million refugees and twenty-six million left homeless.

2

DANGER'S TROUBLED LEGACY: POST-TRAUMATIC STRESS DISORDER

He who would live off war must eventually yield something in return.

— BERTOLT BRECHT

The dangers war journalists work under were exposed, tragically, early on in my study. With the questionnaires en route to him, Miguel Gil Moreno, one of the most respected cameramen in the profession, was killed while covering the civil war in Sierra Leone. Shock, disbelief, outrage, anguish—I would witness these emotions time and again when other war journalists were killed or wounded. That Moreno, who had died a young man, had intimations of his own mortality was revealed in a haunting segment of video interview recorded for a BBC program called *Firing Line*. "The last six years of my life [have been] the most incredible experience a single human being can have," he told the interviewer. "But I cannot see the picture of my family the day they get the phone call saying I have been killed in a war."

Moreno's work as a cameraman brought with it an emotional intensity he was unlikely to experience elsewhere. This explains, in part, his relentless desire to return to areas he knew were hazardous.

And, though he wanted to avoid such issues, in the few lines of that interview he disclosed that he had thought of his passing, no doubt often, given the frequency with which he saw death come to others in his six-year tenure as cameraman to the world's misery. Honored with a Rory Peck Award as freelance cameraperson of the year, Moreno specialized in the visual image, yet ironically the one picture that eluded his imagination was that of his family receiving notification of his death. And that image proved elusive because he could not quite bring himself to believe in it. From this brief insight into his emotional life, we see two competing forces at play. On the one hand we have the images of death and dying that lead to the question, When is it my turn?, a thought so distressing that it can be contemplated only in the abstract. On the other hand, we have avoidance of this thought's logical conclusion, namely the effect on his shocked and grieving family. Moreno stops short of being able to see this tragic denouement; the image is effectively repressed, albeit unconsciously, and as a result he avoids witnessing (and experiencing) the pain and hurt his death will bring to loved ones.

I did not meet Miguel Gil Moreno and must therefore draw back from the temptation of letting an analysis of just two sentences generate an all-embracing clinical opinion. I cannot say whether this intrepid cameraman ever suffered psychologically from what he had seen and experienced, but in that brief, prescient comment captured on film, I find evidence of intrusion and avoidance, two of the three central tenets underpinning a syndrome known as Post-Traumatic Stress Disorder (PTSD).

Much has been written about PTSD, a diagnosis that first appeared in 1980 when the American Psychiatric Association revised its classification system for mental illness. It was not, however, a "new" diagnosis. Earlier variants had included shell shock, combat fatigue and war neurosis. For much of the twentieth century, psychiatrists had recognized that persons who were subjected to life-threatening stressors could decompensate psychologically. What had been contentious was the nature of that decompensation, the signs and symptoms that typically arose in traumatized people. This debate continues to this day, albeit less intensely, with those who believe in the validity of PTSD (a majority) at loggerheads with the skeptics (a minority) who feel the condition has more to do with post-Vietnam psychosocial forces within American society than empirical science. Notwithstanding these rumblings of disquiet, the disorder has been accepted by both the World Health Organization and the American Psychiatric Association as a valid set of symptoms that may follow exposure to a life-threatening stressor.

According to diagnostic criteria, to suffer from PTSD, an individual must have experienced or witnessed an event that involved actual or threatened death or serious injury. Responses to this must involve fear, helplessness or horror. A specified number of symptoms from each of three categories—namely, intrusion, avoidance and arousal—must also be present before the diagnosis can be made. These categories make up the PTSD triad.

Re-experienced or intrusive symptoms include recurrent and involuntary distressing images, thoughts, dreams and flashbacks of the traumatic event. Examples of persistent avoidant symptoms are efforts to ward off thoughts, feelings or conversations associated with the trauma, efforts to stay away from activities, places or people that arouse recollections of the trauma, a restricted range of emotions, a feeling of detachment or estrangement from others and an inability to recall an important aspect of the trauma. Arousal symptoms refer to difficulties with sleep, anger control, concentration, an exaggerated startle response and hypervigilance (such as being wary of potential dangers even when away from a war zone).

There is a consistency to the way people react to catastrophic trauma, irrespective of what the trauma entails. To varying degrees they will persistently re-experience the traumatic event, make attempts to avoid the distressing nature of this involuntary recall and display levels of arousal that affect functions such as sleep and concentration. I assumed the responses the war journalists gave on their questionnaires would show they weren't any different. What I didn't know, however, was how frequently and to what extent they would endorse symptoms of PTSD.

A shared phenomenology should not obscure the manner in which symptoms are acquired. What sets the war journalist apart is a constant need to seek out the conflict, violence and destruction that generate an international headline and without which stories and images are reduced to the blandness of weekly neighborhood reportage. If the threat of peace hangs over every war journalist, however, it is unlikely to occasion more than temporary disappointment. In a world that has consistently shown a rapacious appetite for violence—combined with a diabolical ingenuity for manufacturing it—sustainable peace in many of the world's conflict zones continues to be chimerical. There are always opportunities for war journalists to live willingly in cities under siege, at times subject to the same privations and dangers as the beleaguered residents—getting shot at, wounded, losing friends and colleagues. These experiences play out day after day, the weeks stretching into months and then years. Even soldiers and policemen, to mention two other hazardous professions, operate under a different set of constructs, trying to resolve conflict, not live off its escalation. But events that fizzle out quietly and characters who go peacefully into the night make for dull news. Steve Northup, who photographed the Vietnam War in the mid-1960s for United Press International, said it well when he observed, "When you started out on the day's march, one thing weighed on your mind. If you were going to make really good images that day, something would have to happen; people would have to be hurt or killed. Otherwise, it was just another long, hot walk."

We sat in a small café in the old quarter of Barcelona. It was a winter's afternoon and darkness had come early. I listened to the odyssey of a journalist unfold. In the background the hiss of an espresso machine, the dulcet adagio from a Vivaldi lute concerto and the intermittent staccato of rain on the windowpanes. The man I was interviewing heard none of this. Overwhelmed by memory, he was reliving his years spent in Bosnia. That period in time has never left him. It has defined his life, given him a career, awards, recognition, a livelihood. But there were other things on his mind.

"There are a lot of situations that stay with you. Nightmares. I find myself abusing alcohol and drugs in order not to remember my dreams. In other words, the dreams are there, and if I am on a trip someplace, or go for a week or so without smoking dope or drinking a lot, I find the dreams come back and can be quite disturbing. They are not always there, not every night, but out of a given four or five nights, I might get two or three days of bad sleep and nightmares. And I find that if I go to bed completely stoned and drunk, I can't remember my dreams, so I wake up without having to worry about them. And that for me, in the last few years, has worked, but it's not good, it's not healthy. It screws up many things—your short-term memory, your concentration. I wonder if certain antisocial attitudes that I'm going through over the last few years are related to what's on my mind and how much of those are related to the various drugs and whatnot I am putting into myself to deal with that?"

He paused, looked up, eyes moist, focusing on a point behind me. I was getting toward the end of my series of interviews, and had come to anticipate these moments, a period when the vividness and pain of recall overwhelms speech. I waited patiently for him to go on, for I had also learned that, difficult as it is to recollect the past, the need to talk about it is greater by far.

"I was not feeling well. I wasn't sure of what was wrong with me. I knew it was work related and I knew it was specifically conflict related. So I went to see this fellow for about an hour, in London, and we basically went through everything step by step and he said, 'Well, there is no doubt in my mind you are suffering from PTSD.' And I was quite relieved that somebody had diagnosed what was wrong with me. He gave me some exercises to do, which involved recording the most disturbing episodes in my career, writing them down in a very detailed fashion and then listening to the recordings. He described it as phobia therapy. I did that a few times and found it to be quite effective immediately, but because the therapy wasn't sustained I didn't get better. I was still having nightmares. I remember at the time being sent to a morgue in Egypt to try to find the bodies of some fundamentalists who had been executed. And I remember the smell of the morgue, this disinfectant, this body smell that provoked a very physical reaction in me. I was shaking. I was very emotional, partly because back in Bosnia I'd spent a lot of time in the morgue. The smell of morgues was bad news."

A long pause. The rain stopped and Vivaldi made way for Mozart, the cheerful finale of the fifth violin concerto, the "Turkish." The coffee was replenished. I used the break to summarize what had been said thus far: nightmares, alcohol, cannabis and cocaine to still the dreams, a diagnosis of PTSD, a failure to follow through with therapy, an inability to tolerate the smell of a morgue. I wondered aloud how much more this man had to confide. He told me, with a bitter laugh, that all this was but a prelude.

"I got a bit disgusted with myself. I felt that I was just feeling sorry for myself and that I had to get on with things. So I went to do this war in Yemen, followed by some domestic stories here in Spain, before deciding in early 1995 that I had to go back to Bosnia. I felt it was very important for me to go back to Bosnia. So I did. I had no desire to at all but felt it was an obligation that I had imposed on myself. I felt I had to get back on the horse. I lasted about ten days and I got blown up. A mortar fell fairly close, put a piece of shrapnel into my leg. My flak jacket and equipment stopped other shrapnel. I was operated on in Sarajevo; they gave

me an epidural, pulled out the metal, kept me in hospital for four
or five days and then I was evacuated. Well, can you imagine! In a
sense I had conquered my ghosts, I had gone back, I had overcome
my fear, but I had lasted only ten days before I got blown up. I came
back here to recuperate, and all my friends were saying to me,
'Okay, don't you think that's enough? You've seen this through,
that's enough.' And it was the opposite—I was angry. I was furious.
I had made such a big effort to get back to Sarajevo, such a big effort
to overcome my fears, and now I'm out of the game because some
Serb, a few kilometers away, pops a mortar in on us. Screw that. I'll
carry on. I figured I had invested enough and put enough time and
effort into this at that point that I'd be damned if I was going to
stop. So I carried on."

I was aware there was a war going on, but the battle being fought
was between a man and his personal demons, not between oppos-
ing armies. His fierce determination to use war as a means to con-
quer fear drove this journalist back to the front lines. The desire to
report the news, to get the breaking story, was still there, but for the
moment it was displaced as a priority. The challenge was vintage
Hemingway, and it seemed apt that this self-administered test was
being discussed in the land that is home to the bullfight. But comparisons between a matador sweating the big drop and war journalism are of course specious, for the outcome in war is far less
certain than the one handed out in the late-afternoon corrida. The
man who sat in front of me, giving vent to his frustrations, fears and
anger, had lost his way in a dangerous profession. War had sapped
his emotional and physical resources, and yet it was to war that
he went looking to replenish them. By now my curiosity as a
researcher had given way to the concerns of a clinician. The odyssey
was not yet complete, but the ending was disturbingly predictable.

"It has come to the point that I no longer want to go out. I do
not want to meet people. If my partner goes away for a weekend,
I lock myself up in the house and order in food and just stay drunk
and stoned. I have become a recluse. I do not want to deal with

people. I have become hyperaware, hyperalert to noises and other such things that bother me. But on a social level, I do not want any new experiences."

In this vignette are to be found all the cardinal features of post-traumatic stress disorder. There are the unwanted, traumatic memories that return as nightmares or are triggered by a certain smell. There is the hypervigilance and difficulty concentrating. And finally there is reclusive behavior and substance abuse, both attempts at numbing or damping down the painful recollections. In my interviews with the war journalists I found that 29 percent of the group met the diagnostic criteria for PTSD.

A notable observation here was that PTSD symptoms were differentially distributed according to the type of journalism practiced. Thus, symptoms were more frequent and intense in stills photographers; they were followed by cameramen and then print reporters and producers. The necessity for proximity to an event —encapsulated in the Hungarian photographer Robert Capa's famous dictum, "If your photographs are not good enough, you are not close enough—" offers the most parsimonious explanation for these findings. Across all domains of war journalism, the overall PTSD lifetime rate of 29 percent well exceeds the rate of 5 percent in the general population and 7 to 13 percent for traumatized policemen. It comes close to that reported in combat veterans and (depending on the veteran's degree of combat exposure) may, in certain cases, exceed it.*

While these comparisons are informative, they obscure another fundamental difference between war journalism and other hazardous professions: policemen, firefighters and soldiers are schooled in violence and danger. They enter their workplace with the expectation of encountering them and are trained over months or years to learn how to deal with them. Journalists have little of this prepa-

---

* None of the domestic journalists in the control group were diagnosed with PTSD.

ration. The typical war journalist is someone who, after leaving college or university, drifts into conflict zones either by design or, more often, by chance, unprepared for the dangers ahead. For some, the harsh realities of war prove too unsettling. After covering one or two conflicts, they move on to other work. Those who stay are exposed to repetitive cycles of danger while working and safety when back home, and such are the extremes represented by these states that, for some, both may prove psychologically enervating.

Even among the more than 70 percent of journalists who do not have the full PTSD syndrome, isolated intrusive symptoms persist and prove troubling. One journalist who had covered the wars in Bosnia and Chechnya and who felt he had coped well with both, nevertheless found his behavior changed on his return to London. "Coming back from Bosnia, I had a funny feeling every time I walked on grass. I just avoided grass for fear of landmines in Bosnia. I still have that feeling—if I am walking on the pavement and have to step off onto some grass, I become a little agitated."

For a journalist who had reported on the genocide in Rwanda, the slaughter and mounds of corpses lived with him seven years later, intruding into his consciousness with an unpredictability that was disconcerting. "I think the images and smells and experiences stayed with me for months because of their intensity," he told me. "Remember, I had been through a lot of conflicts before that, but this was on a dramatically different scale. I was back about a week, and my wife and I were invited to a friend's house in north London. As I lifted a drink to my lips, there was the smell of corpses from the glass of champagne. I just had to put it down. That has happened a lot, the sense that the smell was all over you, that no matter how many times you washed your clothes, it would not go away."

For this journalist, therapy had helped with some of the more troubling recollections but had been unable to halt the demons that came intermittently with sleep, stealing into his dreams when his guard was down. "The most common dream I had was being trapped under a mound of bodies and not being able to get out. And then there was another variation to this, in which I was trapped under this mound of bodies and a guy above with a machete was trying to get down to kill me."

For another journalist, the dreams seldom came while he was working. "If I have been on a hard job and have seen a lot of violence, as in Chechnya, for example, I won't usually have any dreams. It seems that when I get back home, I start having two or three a week. In these dreams there is a lot of mutilation, a lot of darkness and a lot of fear, but they are not direct replicas of what I have seen. They are more abstract and might be of dismembered bodies and disemboweled bodies, but not actually what I have seen."

While intrusive symptoms tend to decrease over time, for the majority of the 140 war journalists studied, they never disappeared entirely. During the period I collected my data, the first Chechen war was already over, the Balkans had gone quiet and the Middle East had yet to erupt. Only regional African conflicts, such as those in Sierra Leone, the Congo and Angola, continued with their unrelenting pattern of massacre and mutilation. Most war journalists were between traumas, with many weeks, if not months, since their last exposure to danger. Yet despite this lull in hostilities, 62 percent still reported unwanted recollections of traumatic events, 77 percent described flashbacks and a similar percentage experienced strong and unpleasant waves of emotion associated with involuntarily recollections. Thus, even those journalists without PTSD experienced isolated, persistent and at times disturbing, intrusive symptoms.

Experience offers little protection from these symptoms. Whether a neophyte or veteran, the journalist often pays a terrible price in his search for a conflict's defining image. Dan Eldon was a twenty-two-year-old photojournalist on his first assignment for Reuters when he was stoned to death by an enraged mob in Somalia. Two of his Reuters colleagues, Anthony Macharia and Hos Maina and a colleague from Associated Press, Hansi Kraus, suffered the same fate. Eldon kept a series of journals, which were documented after his death in *Dying to Tell the Story*, a film by his mother, Kathy, and sister Amy. In one, Eldon writes that "the terror of being surrounded by violence and the horrors of the famine threw me into a dark depression. Even journalists who had covered many conflicts were moved to tears. But for me, this was my first experience with war. Before Somalia, I had only seen two dead bodies in my life. Now I have seen hundreds, tossed into ditches like sacks. The worst things I could not photograph." After one particularly difficult stint he confides, "It was a horrible and terrifying experience. . . . Being in a place like that really eats away at the mind. . . . When I left I had gone a little nuts. . . . I don't know how these experiences have changed me, but I feel different."

In her quest to find out what happened to her brother on that hot, violent afternoon in Mogadishu, Amy Eldon sought out others in the profession, including Don McCullin, one of the great war photojournalists. For her film, she interviewed him in a gallery exhibiting his work. The black-and-white prints are startling, the faces and bodies of soldiers, civilians, children saturated with anguish. It is unsettling to see these images, for they force us to open our eyes and minds and confront a nightmare existence. What, then, do they say of the man who took the pictures? For decades, Don McCullin has pushed his lens into the face of grief, despair, hopelessness, misery. He may have been able to retreat to the comfort of his home in England at periodic intervals, but it is clear this has not kept the demons at bay. The cumulative weight of all that sadness has left its psychological imprint. In *Dying to Tell the Story*, Don McCullin appears melancholic, a recluse haunted by the images lining the walls of the gallery. He tells Amy Eldon, "Emotionally I was like a destroyed person." Those images, which have brought him fame, will not let him be, their memory a constant companion. A collection of his most famous photographs is entitled *Sleeping with Ghosts: A Life's Work in Photography* and the title speaks to the repetitive, intrusive nature of his traumatic memories. He imagines a ghoulish spectacle unfolding each night in his home, a morbid variant of *Coppelia*, in which the ghosts of the victims he has photographed come together in a macabre meeting of departed souls.

Mohammed Shaffi, a Reuters cameraman who accompanied her brother that fateful afternoon, also agreed to be interviewed by Amy Eldon. Although badly beaten, Shaffi alone survived the mob's frenzied attack, and his account is therefore central to understanding the events surrounding his colleagues' deaths. Four years have passed since the stoning, and he has returned to the scene of the killing, accompanied by Amy Eldon. "I can't forget what has happened," he confides emotionally into the camera. Tears come easily and, like Don McCullin, he too seems subdued by the weight of cumulative memory.

A few years after *Dying to Tell the Story* was aired, Mohammed Shaffi wrote to me. "My big problem is I cannot sleep. I still get flashbacks of the stories I had covered, people being killed in front of my eyes in their hundreds. I can see myself running while bullets are flying over my head. The truth is, I am afraid to sleep. I talk a lot in my sleep. The next morning I can remember everything I had gone through the night before. I love my work, and nothing will or can stop me covering hard-news stories. When I am alone my mind goes back to what I have gone through. I feel sick and very tired. I have never spoken to my family about this because I don't want them to worry."

His reference to his family reminded me of something he said in Kathy Eldon's film. "The work I was doing was more important than my family," he admits. "I have the rest of my life to make it up to them." In that, however, he was mistaken. Six months after I received his letter, Mohammed Shaffi was found dead in a hotel room in Jerusalem. He had had a heart attack. He was fifty years old.

———

The florid nature of the dreams, the eidetic quality of recall, the power of the past to intrude repetitively into the present or constantly, involuntarily reinvent itself makes for dramatic narrative. These symptoms come to define whether a person has become psychologically distressed, and while they may be considered the quintessential feature of PTSD, they may not prove the most disabling. Time may diminish their frequency and intensity, but for many war journalists, they never completely disappear, insinuating themselves into the mental fabric of existence, disconcerting, albeit no longer terrifying.

Not so the avoidance phenomena, the second group of symptoms that make up the PTSD triad. These occur frequently, and the most prevalent of all is a feeling of detachment or estrangement from other people. Not surprisingly, the effect on relationships is often destructive. One camerawoman echoed the sentiments of many of her colleagues when she said, "While I was doing the Croatia-Bosnia stuff, I was out in the field all the time. And I was moving around. I'd be one of the guys. I'd be living in army barracks and stuff like that. Then I'd get back home, and someone would invite me to a dinner party, and people would be talking about Bernie's car or skiing holidays in Switzerland and I'd feel like I was not fitting in. I would sit there thinking, You guys don't know anything about the real world. It got so that I did not want to see these people, and they had been my friends. I do that even now. Last weekend, I didn't go out at all. I just did not feel like it."

War journalists are acutely aware of the contrast between the intensity of living and working in a war zone and the mundaneness of life in a society at peace. No matter the conflict, a couple of hours in a plane will have you back in London or Paris in a comfortable bed in a quiet apartment, the stores stocked with every imaginable item, people laughing and carefree, caught up in the rhythm of life in a civil society. Details like paying the electricity bill or getting the lawn cut, when placed alongside death and survival, heroism and cowardice, can seem annoyingly trivial. A wedge is inserted between two disparate realities, the world inhabited by war journalists and their coterie of soldiers, refugees, mercenaries, informants, fixers, and that occupied by the journalists' families with their shopkeepers, schoolteachers, appliance repairmen and garage attendants. The adjustment for journalists when they re-enter this orbit poses a challenge, and it can test their emotional maturity and the strength of their relationships.

The French photojournalist Jerome Delay told me the story of coming home from his first trip to Sarajevo. "We had difficulty getting out of the city. I was with a *Washington Post* correspondent. There was a lot of fighting going on, and we waited for an hour, two hours, three hours. Then at one point we said, 'Okay, let's go for it.' So I put on two flak jackets and drove up to the Bosnian checkpoint. 'Is the road okay?' I asked, and the soldier said, 'Well, it might be.' So we hit it. There's a stretch of road about three kilometers long. We picked up speed, passed a burned-out truck, took a sharp right turn, came under fire but made it through. I spent the night in Split, got drunk, got on a plane to Frankfurt, got drunk in Frankfurt at nine in the morning. Then I flew to London. All of a sudden I was alone in this plane and then in Heathrow. I took a cab to a hotel. The cab driver wanted to talk and I told her, 'Listen, I'm sorry, but I don't want to talk, so just shut up.' And we drove through these London suburbs to go downtown and I saw people who were not running. There were all these . . . all these shops. . . . It was dark. It was raining. Food everywhere. Food. It was overwhelming, the quantity of things. It was almost . . . not insane, it was disgusting, and there is one thing I wanted to do from then on. It was just to go back. Because I felt . . . it was not normal. My normalcy was no running water, people running, and shelling. That was where I had become comfortable. That was my reality. Then I went to this hotel and spent two days there, just doing nothing, not seeing anybody, and then I came home. I have learned not to come straight home. Because every time I have done it, it has not been good."

Delay even came up against the everyday challenges of life away from a war zone while he was in Bosnia. "I remember talking to my wife on my cell phone while I was in Sarajevo, and she tells me, 'Oh, we've got a big problem. The washing machine is not working properly.' I go, 'Honey, excuse me, but we have not had running water here for two and a half months, okay? So, I don't know ... buy a new machine, have it fixed. I really don't care.' Later I realized that was really the wrong thing to say, because their world is very important. They have their parameters and I have mine too, when I'm away on assignment. We each have our markers, and one thing I've learned over the years is to respect those markers. And yes, to my wife and two little girls, the fact that the washing machine was not working was as important to them as the absence of running water was to me in Sarajevo. My wife respected me more than I respected her in that regard."

For journalists based in Europe, the Bosnian war was literally on their doorstep. They could spend the morning under siege in Sarajevo and the afternoon taking a stroll in the Ramblas or Tuileries. The temporal proximity of London, Paris or Madrid to war heightened the sense of unreality attached to the whole conflict. It seemed barely credible that a war accompanied by ethic cleansing and concentration camps could take root on European soil yet again. And innovative technology and the unprecedented ease of communication only added to the general befuddlement. During a lull in the shelling, a journalist could reach for a cell phone and contact an editor, a spouse, friend, lover. Hunkered down in some ruined church or deserted basement journalists would run up against the blandness of domestic life back home. Not all welcomed such reminders.

Finding a middle ground that acknowledges two distinct realities often proves elusive. When journalists return home from war, their sense of estrangement may be matched by their partner's trouble fathoming what life is like in a conflict zone. An effort to appear understanding, to shield the war journalist from events that are perceived as trivial, may upset the equilibrium of a relationship. The partner who stays home can abrogate his or her sense of identity, subscribing to a view of life that equates war with meaning and relegates everything outside of war to the boring and unremarkable. This folie à deux becomes, in time, untenable. Relationships wither.

When it comes to making the transition from a conflict zone to civil society, few have traveled the route more often than James Nachtwey. The celebrated American photographer has not missed a war in twenty years. His professional longevity is a source of admiration and wonder to colleagues who see him as the standard-bearer of a tradition in war photography going back to such icons as Larry Burrows, Robert Capa and Eugene Smith. Nachtwey, the subject of an Academy Award–nominated documentary, *War Photographer*, was not an easy man to get hold of. For more than half the year he is away from home, mostly working in areas of conflict. When we did finally meet, I found observing the man to be almost as interesting as listening to what he had to say. Of slight build, he has an immaculate appearance but dresses very simply. The fastidiousness—precise, neat, unruffled, no stray lock of hair or trace of stubble—reflects an understated persona. His apartment—restrained, orderly, elegant—mirrors his personal appearance. His voice, too, is revealing—a quiet, measured monotone with minimal emotional inflection, or what neurologists term prosody. A temperate manner of speaking, without mannerism or gesture matches the delivery. The overall impression is of an aesthete, the tranquillity, orderliness, restraint a foil to the inferno captured by his camera.

When he was younger Nachtwey's sense of disconnection from life back home was similar to that of his current colleagues. "At first I thought people were spoiled and they had too much and how could they possibly be concerned about such petty things," he told me. But in time, his perspective underwent a metamorphosis: the angry denunciation was turned inside out. "I think my early views were immature and inexperienced," he explained, "because after a couple of years I actually was glad that those petty things were all that people had to be concerned about. I was very happy for them. I'm really happy that's what they have to deal with. That they don't have to deal with having family members killed in front of their eyes, and having their houses destroyed and their culture destroyed and being oppressed. This is what normal life is and people do get worried about things that, compared to the enormity of where I have just been, can seem petty and foolish. But I actually hope the worst thing that ever happens to them is that their cab didn't show up on time or something. And I am actually grateful that's the case."

But Nachtwey is the exception. The sense of estrangement many journalists feel on their return from war and the difficulties this introduces into relationships translate into a high percentage of unmarried war journalists. Of those I studied, over half were either single or divorced. The comparable figure for domestic journalists who have never been to war is one-third unattached, a difference that is statistically highly significant. Even more illuminating are the statistics from the population at large: by the time a person reaches his or her fifth decade (remember the average age of the war journalists is about forty years), the large majority are married.

While emotional detachment is psychologically crippling for some war journalists, it was not the most striking symptom of avoidant behavior that I encountered. More dramatic was the inability to remember an important aspect of a traumatic event, evidence of the power of the mind to censor memory. One television cameraman displayed this when he related to me an experience in Somalia in 1993. "One day we were in Mogadishu—in one of those communication vehicles with a driver and two armed guards in the back—in the midst of a very large crowd outside the American embassy. They started to try to drag me out of the car. They were all going mad. A lot of gunmen were around us, and we drove right through the crowd. Then I'm not sure what happened, but there was gunfire—we were shooting all over the place and I was being pulled out of the car. My only memory I really have of that time is seeing a marine behind the gates of the embassy just looking away and not doing anything. I also vaguely remember trying to get my sunglasses back from some guy. So I am not sure how many people we killed, if we killed any, that is, and how many we ran over. I have no real memory of that."

Detachment, estrangement, amnesia—all are common symptoms of avoidance reported by the war journalists. However, one symptom seldom gets mentioned, and that is the effort to evade thoughts, feelings or conversations associated with the trauma. Here the war journalists are in a unique bind, for it is that central traumatic event that often constitutes the news. The print reporter, in preparing her story, will have to revisit in her mind what has occurred. Memory is essential to the process; without it there is no story. Similarly, the television reporter or cameraman will have to pore over the images captured on film, until the story has been visually conveyed to his satisfaction. The nature of this bind is now revealed; the demands of the profession are at odds with how an individual may respond to overwhelming stressors. This tension between job obligation and personal response may not necessarily be a bad thing, however, for in being forced to confront the traumatic event, repeatedly if necessary, war journalists are given a cathartic outlet, an opportunity to work through and process on both a cognitive and an emotional level what has befallen them. But to the less resilient among them, this constant revisiting of past traumas may upset an already fragile emotional equilibrium, driving them further into a tightly cocooned, emotionally constricted existence. "It slowly takes away your smile" is the way Joao Silva describes it.

———

The final part of the PTSD triad are symptoms of arousal, which include difficulties with sleep, irritability or temper outbursts and poor concentration. These symptoms are not specific to PTSD sufferers, for they are found in many people with psychiatric disorders and, to lesser degrees, in the population at large. Of all the arousal symptoms, the two most significant are hypervigilance and an exaggerated startle response. Both were frequently experienced by war journalists.

The following anecdote, related to me by a BBC reporter, illustrates how the threat of danger in a war zone follows the journalist home. "Once, when I was in the middle of covering the Bosnian war, I went down to visit a good friend who happens to be a journalist as well as a political correspondent in London," he told me. "He lives in a village in Hampshire, and we went out for a walk on a beautiful, crisp Sunday morning. He has a little boy, about four years old at the time, and he went with us. We were walking along a tarmac road, thinking or talking about nothing connected with work. Suddenly the little boy spotted something and ran up a grassy verge and my heart leaped. I ran after him and shouted, 'No, no, no, don't go there!' I was thinking of landmines, just coming off the tarmac. It was absurd."

A cameraman just returned from the charnel house of Grozny reported a similar experience. "You'd have the twitches, you know," he confided, "and I could never forget it. Shortly after coming back to England, I was filming at the Paddington Green police station. The police had a couple of suspects, and the press wanted to film them. I was just standing there and a lorry drove over a plastic bottle and it sort of exploded, and you have never seen anyone hit the deck so quickly. And everyone just looked at me and said, 'God, what's wrong with you?'"

The startle response is often accompanied by other symptoms of arousal, most often irritability. One journalist told me the story of a going-away party he attended soon after returning from Zaire. "I had come straight from the airport, dumped my bags and gone off to have this drink session," he recalled. "Literally within a day, you come back from a war zone to London and you are off to a TGIF place where they had all these balloons for the party. Somebody popped a balloon and I was down on the floor before I realized it. The people around me knew I had been out in the field, but the waiter thought it would be funny to pop some more balloons and see my reaction. As I said, my aggression levels were right up there, and it's like 'Whew!' I was on my way over to him and the waiter wasn't too sure what was going on and I was diverted by three of four of my mates, straight out the door. Yeah, it's important to have friends who understand the situation."

Yet despite reactions like these and the others I have described, it would be misleading to convey the impression that war journalists are riddled with PTSD-type psychopathology. There is no doubt that the risks they expose themselves to are astonishing by whatever standards, for at times, in their eagerness to capture the news of war, they place themselves in the vanguard of armies. But what is perhaps more extraordinary is that over 70 percent do not have PTSD. Every account of unwanted intrusive thoughts, nightmares, startle responses and emotional withdrawal was matched by a story of journalists taken to the brink of death in the most perverse and sadistic fashion, yet reacting with equanimity. Certain people appear immune to the long-term, adverse psychological consequences of repeated exposure to life-threatening danger. This is not to say they never experience fear, but rather that their threshold for it is raised, their emotional responses more circumscribed and transient.

"A colleague and I were covering an offensive," one photographer told me of his Balkan experiences. "We were arrested by the Serbs. It seemed initially like a routine arrest—I didn't think much of it. Then something must have happened, because the tension level went up much higher. We got handcuffed, thrown into a car, driven off to some remote location, and there we were interrogated, separated, beaten, hoods were placed over our heads and we were subjected to mock executions. I was being held in a wooden shed. They left me in there, but took my colleague out. A gun went off and a few minutes later they came back and took me into another room where there was this commander, and they told me they had just executed my friend and that if I did not confess to being a spy in the next hour, they would execute me too."

While he talked I observed the man closely. There were no outward signs of emotion. He paused, took a sip of a Diet Coke and resumed his dispassionate account.

"I had nothing to confess, so I did not do anything. I said I was a photographer and stuck to the story. The hood was placed over my head again, my hands, which were now uncuffed, were tied behind my back and I was taken into another room. They asked me, 'What is your mission here?' I said I was a photographer. This went on for about fifteen minutes or so. Each time I answered they would punch me in the face. They accused us of being spies and said we were there illegally, which we were not. It was very cold and they had doused us with water, so it was very uncomfortable and my main thought was to keep warm and all the while I was replaying things in my mind, trying to figure out whether what they had said was true. I had not heard my colleague call out after the shot had gone off, I had not heard a body fall, so had they really shot him?"

I had this man's questionnaires in front of me, and I glanced again at his PTSD responses. For each question the respondent can choose one of five options: not at all, a little bit, moderately, quite a bit and extremely. In this case a neat tick had been placed in the "not at all" column for twenty of the twenty-two PTSD questions. The remaining two were rated "a little bit."

"I had become very calm and very clear-headed and also very accepting of the inevitable—that I was ready for them. Whether I would have felt that way when they put the gun to my head, I don't know, but I really felt I was ready to accept my fate."

He took another sip of Diet Coke. I commented on what an ordeal it must have been and asked whether he felt fear at any point. "Yeah, yeah, I was scared, but I was not scared in a hysterical way. One thing that I did do, that I had learned, I guess, from previous experience, was that it was not wise to be completely calm in front of them because they would think you were a real professional spy, as it were. So I kind of acted more outwardly scared when I was with them, hoping to make them feel sorry for me, or something like that."

As I listened to this account of horrendous maltreatment, I was reminded of two researchers, Holmes and Rahe, who had, back in the 1980s, devised a rating scale that quantified life events. Points were assigned to changing a job, getting married, the death of a family member, moving house and so on. The more stressful the event, the more points were awarded. The aim of the whole exercise was to show that if someone's points exceeded a certain threshold within a finite period, say the past six months or a year, his or her chances of developing a psychiatric illness would be significantly increased. What, I wondered, would Holmes and Rahe have made of this man's experience? Held captive, isolated, freezing, wet, hooded, handcuffed, repeatedly punched, his colleague presumably executed, facing a similar fate within the hour. His score is off the chart. It cannot be quantified. And what is his response? Of all things, he has to simulate fear, not control it.

The story does not end there, for there is an addendum that shifts a remarkable narrative into the realm of the fantastic. The war journalist waited to the very end of his story to reveal that all his tribulations at the hands of his captors were superimposed on another more alarming fact. "Everybody has gone through this type of thing, to varying degrees, all the way to actually getting killed. But I had seen a number of executions in front of me, by Serbs against Croatians and Bosnians, and I had photographed some of them, which caused more trouble for me with them. Some people were looking for me. A price had been placed on my head by a warlord-paramilitary-mafia guy and I was very worried that the Serbs holding me would make the connection between me and this warlord."

There were multiple layers of trauma to be peeled away here, and like an archaeologist seeking hidden truths, I went looking for the man submerged within. One by one, traumatic events were revealed, carefully defined and their essential characteristics clarified before they were put to one side and we moved on to the next layer. Eventually, all the threats, dousings, humiliations, beatings and mock executions administered over the course of a five-year conflict were cataloged. And when all this had been done, what emotional residue was left? The answer is very little. The man does not have PTSD. He is not depressed. He does not drink excessively. He does not use drugs. He loves his work. Yes, at times, he has been frightened, but never for long.

Are we to express incredulity or admiration? Are the responses of this journalist no more than those of a naysayer, unable to disentangle himself from the macho image of his profession? Would an admission of fearful nightmares or startle responses shatter a carefully constructed persona? In the end, I came to reject these possibilities. The relative absence of psychological distress was not unique to him. Others responded in a similar fashion to stressors equally severe. One was Elizabeth Jones, a Canadian freelance camerawoman.

"The worst situation I had was in Kisangani, in the north of the Congo, in 1997. There were a lot of Interahamwe around Kisangani because the Rwandan refugee camps were being broken up. There were a few journalists in town—we all knew each other and were staying at the same hotel. There was a cameraman at one of the big news agencies, and he was collecting all of our tapes to take them to the airport and ship them out. He got to the airport and somebody recognized him from an earlier episode in the war and thought he was a Belgian mercenary because he had a crew cut and did look like one. The airport was absolutely full, with thousands of soldiers who were retreating. And they just opened fire on him. He survived actually, but a number of people around him were killed. I was not actually there for any of this. He was rescued from this hail of bullets by a couple of guys who threw him into their car and drove him to the edge of the airport, where they stuck a gun to his head and said, 'Give us everything you've got. How much money do you have?' And he had, maybe $10 so he said he did not have much, but a friend of his over at the mission had a lot of money. That was me, and so at this point I was completely oblivious to what was going on.

"What happened next was that I was at the mission and these nutty guys with guns came raging into the room, with a gun to the head of this guy and other guns blazing away. It was very scary and they said, 'Who is the woman with the money? Which one? Is that you?' And pointed at me. I leaped behind a door. I thought they were going to shoot me. It was a very ugly moment. . . . I do not know how long it lasted, but they were really threatening everybody else at the mission as well—pointing guns and then they just grabbed my camera and gear, and I threw the money out of my wallet and gave them all I had—which was quite a lot—and they stormed out with this guy and I assumed they had taken him off to be shot. We did not know what to do. I was with a colleague of that cameraman and he just collapsed. He completely broke down. He did not know what to do."

It has been interesting to observe the war journalists during their interviews. The notes I made, essentially a record of their mental state at the time, were often as informative as what they themselves had to say. During our interview, Jones was sitting on a settee with her feet drawn up under her. She was attractive, relaxed, calm, brow unfurrowed, at ease with herself and the story she was relating. To me, the outside observer, there was an incongruity between her exterior equanimity and the turbulent events of her narrative. I reminded myself that the Congo is this woman's passion, a land she has returned to many times, always alone, to make critically acclaimed, self-financed, money-losing documentaries about a country the size of France, Germany, Italy, Britain and Spain combined, a country that few in the West are interested in.

Congo. There is no country in Africa with a more evocative name. Africa's impenetrable, ungovernable heart, dark, foreboding, a metaphor for chaos. It is this caldron that the woman I was interviewing had chosen as her workplace. Every day she rubbed shoulders with genocidal Interahamwe, rogue militias, ill-disciplined armies, mercenaries and displaced millions, while confronting the risk of cholera, AIDS, yellow fever and malaria, among the more pernicious health hazards. In this malignant climate of death and disease, events unfold at speed and with unpredictability. Her story was testimony to that. It also demonstrated a temperament that soaks up adversity.

"I was feeling fine, actually," she said, picking up the threads of her story, "although I knew I was really being tested. It was a most frightening moment, and these guys were ready to kill. They were pointing their guns up your nose and were very threatening in a loud, aggressive, blow-your-brains-out kind of way. It was really horrible—they had disappeared with the cameraman, and we did not know if they were going to shoot him and then come back for us. His colleague just freaked out—he was in tears, a real basket case. I was thinking to myself that I felt quite okay. I was conscious of the fact that I was able to make decisions. When I have been put into that sort of situation I often think that I am more calm than the other people around me. So it must be something within me."

This last statement was said in the most matter-of-fact way, without a trace of bravura. She has been in tough situations, seen the reactions of some of her male colleagues and judged her responses against theirs. She was unable to articulate these differences, other than to say there is something within her, some poorly understood characteristic that allows her to deal calmly with terror. But this is no foolhardy trait, as the ending to her story shows.

"I went outside the mission to see if the militia were going to shoot this cameraman, and at that moment a truckful of soldiers pulled up and arrested me and the other guy, who was still crying. They then went around the town picking up all the journalists they could find and threw us all into some kind of holding room. The whole episode lasted twenty-four hours. I was separated from the men, as I was the only woman, and some of the men were beaten.

I was just kept alone, so I did not know whether they were planning to rape me. I had no idea what was going on, but I was thinking clearly and one thing that I had done at the mission was rather clever, for I had found a priest and told him to phone the British consulate, which he did. That had been a good thing to do, because there was no other opportunity to tell people what had happened to us. The twenty-four hours passed slowly. I was just bored and hungry and thirsty. Eventually we were taken to the secret service headquarters and given a long lecture. We were then given a car with a driver who was supposed to take us back to the hotel, but it all ended rather comically, as it can in the Congo, when the car ran out of gas. We were all dispatched to find some petrol in the middle of the night, so we all ended walking back to our hotel."

Shaken up by this episode, she took a break from Africa. A year later, however, she was back in the Congo.

———

There is a clearly discernible thread that runs through all the war journalists' responses. Whether they reported symptoms of PTSD or not, they share a belief that their work has changed them. Here, it is informative to cite Chris Hedges's book, *War Is a Force That Gives Us Meaning*. After three harrowing trips to the civil war in El Salvador, Hedges finally left the country under considerable emotional strain. "My last act was, in a frenzy of rage and anguish, to leap over the KLM counter in the airport in Costa Rica because of a perceived slight by a hapless airline clerk. I beat him to the floor as his bewildered colleagues locked themselves in the room behind the counter. Blood streamed down his face and mine. I refused to wipe the dried stains off my cheeks on the flight to Madrid, and I carry a scar on my face from where he thrust his pen into my cheek. War's sickness had become mine." This overwrought behavior comes not from some paparazzo with psychopathic tendencies but from a respected journalist with a stellar pedigree—foreign correspondent to the *New York Times* for over a decade; part of a Pulitzer Prize–winning team; an adjunct professor of journalism at New York University; holder of a bachelor of arts degree from Colgate University, a master's in divinity from Harvard University and a Nieman Fellowship, also at Harvard. The jarring dissonance of a divinity major hurdling the check-in counter to assault an airline attendant is matched by the very public emotional disintegration of the ITN cameraman Jon Steele at Heathrow's Terminal 4. His memoir, *War Junkie*, opens with savage self-deprecation. "Attention, Club World and World Traveller passengers. British Airways is happy to announce the nervous breakdown of Jon Denis Steele, at check-in counter twenty."

If such public manifestations of distress are uncommon, the underlying emotions are not. The many personal anecdotes given to me are testimony to that. When I looked beyond the scotomatous domain of symptom checklists and structured psychiatric interviews, the war journalists I met, to a man and woman, spoke about the ability of remarkable events to move them to tears, anger, rage, euphoria, frustration, hatred, love. Such were the magnitude of these events and the intensity of emotions generated that they would never again view their world as before. To varying degrees, this translated into an awakened or bolstered social conscience mixed, at times, with embitterment and deep cynicism. Once you have viewed the world through the prism of war, your perspective on life invariably alters.

Throughout this chapter the voices of the journalists themselves have illustrated the ways that war has profoundly affected them. It is therefore fitting that the final word on the subject goes to one of their most articulate spokesmen, the BBC's Allan Little, who reported in the *Evening Standard* that a feisty exchange among war journalists took place in London at a meeting where I presented my data to the profession.

"The historian Philip Knightley, who has written a brilliant book on war correspondents, was also there on Thursday night,"

Little wrote. "He recited, with some condescension, a canon of war correspondent 'greats,' such as Alexander Clifford, Alan White-head, Martha Gellhorn and Ernest Hemingway. What, he mused, would they have made of all this self-indulgent talk of trauma? I think this question was designed to intimidate or shame us. Well, I am neither intimidated nor shamed. For I have seen a lot of war and I think I know what it can do. Do you not think Hemingway broached this subject? Why do we do this? Why do we love it? What are we obsessed with, living so dangerously, drinking so heavily, bursting into tears so easily? Oh yes [he] did!"

After urging his fellow war journalists to take responsibility for their actions and avoid a compensation culture, reminding them that in relation to the victims of war their difficulties are insignificant, Little ended with this simple caution: "Do not delude yourself into thinking that you can swan in and out of other people's wars year after year and not be affected in some way."

3

WHY TAKE THE RISKS?

I could never say I've had enough wars. If I did, maybe my brain would stop functioning.

— PETER ARNETT

"WAR IN EUROPE OVER. There is absolutely no reason to get up in the mornings any more." So ends the memoir of Robert Capa, the great war photographer. A revealing final statement and one that encapsulates a philosophy of life that is shared by many of his colleagues. War may be "that stupid crime, that devil's madness," yet for a small group of men and women, and they number no more than a couple of hundred, it acts like a magnet, attracting them to environs often far-flung, always dangerous, and in the process conferring meaning on their lives and making it that much easier to get up in the morning and face each day.

Why should this be? Why is it that war journalists return repeatedly to scenes of carnage and suffering, placing themselves at great personal risk, venturing into areas that have regularly and disturbingly claimed the lives of colleagues and friends? Perhaps in the case of those journalists who are untroubled psychologically by their work, such behavior is a little easier to fathom. But what they all share, irrespective of whether they have one or two symptoms of PTSD or the full-blown disorder, is a relentless drive to tell the story of war. For many of the veterans, those who have been in the field for a decade or more, the intermittent nightmares, flashbacks and moodiness are seldom deterrents. Colleagues are buried, friends are mourned and still they return to the fray. Even the death of eight journalists in post–September 11, 2001, Afghanistan in little over a week failed to drive them from the battlefield. At times, this tenacity in the face of so much horror and personal loss perplexes the journalists themselves. Fergal Keane, mourning the loss of his BBC colleague John Harrison in the Bantustans of South Africa in 1994, wrote bitterly, "Journalists race around in search of civil war, secretly happiest when they sign off from some hell hole where the bodies are stacking up and the omens of apocalypse are most vivid. I am sick to the teeth of war stories, the flak jackets and all the attendant bullshit. Why did we do it all? Why do people like John and me and countless others race around townships and battle zones? I am still searching for the answer, but I know that pursuit of the truth is only one part of the equation."

Even before I began my interviews with war journalists, I often heard the term "adrenaline junkie" bandied about by those who were acquainted with the profession. The difficulty with the term, however, is that while it has some biochemical legitimacy, it also has pejorative, demeaning undertones. Still, not everyone is sensitive to the connotations. The ITN cameraman Jon Steele openly acknowledged the addictive quality of danger in the provocative title of his memoir, *War Junkie*. Notwithstanding Steele's cri de coeur account, many war journalists find the term offensive because it conjures up an image of behavior enslaved to violence, of a base craving for a fix, devoid of personal choice, intellectual curiosity or morality. Their actions thus appear inherently selfish, the journalists using war and the catastrophic misery of others as a vehicle for fulfilling their own egotistic needs.

Many war journalists have looked inward and readily admit to the high that comes from experiencing and surviving combat, for even if their role on the battlefield is that of observer, the dangers they face are often no different from those confronted by combatants. Although the majority admitted to a rush of excitement that buoys them during or following combat, they all insisted their motivation extended beyond attaining a state of exhilarated physiological arousal.

Yet despite these disclaimers, war as a stimulant was one of the themes that ran through the interviews I obtained. Fergal Keane recalled that "what I got out of war was a buzz. You don't ever feel more alive. You know the shelling is going on and you are exposed to this intense experience and at the time it seems like the most important thing in the world. It's just so addictive. So addictive."

Jeremy Bowen spoke of going to "places I knew would be dangerous, and it troubled me at the time. I had several, probably half a dozen, experiences when I thought, I am going to die. Fucking hell, I have really had it. And there were many, many other times where the bullets were whizzing all over the place and I suddenly got this feeling, what have I done? What have I done? What the hell am I doing here? But that feeling would subside when we got the story. Yet again I wasn't dead. I was alive, and that was for a while, in a strange way, exhilarating."

Bowen perfectly captures the invigorating effects of life in a war zone. "It was a very intense experience," he explained to me. "After a day in Sarajevo, or one of the other places, the colors would seem brighter, drink would taste better, you would get excited." With this account of heightened visual and gustatory sensation, one can appreciate that for Bowen, life away from a war zone was at times hard. "In the mid nineties, when Sarajevo was going on, I loved it and hated not being there. I had terrible withdrawal symptoms when I left." The challenges of readjusting to life back in peaceful England became even greater when he decided to leave war journalism. "It has actually been a very difficult transition for me, really difficult," he explained. "I still have many doubts. Eight days after I left the Middle East, the current cycle of violence kicked off in Jerusalem and I wasn't there.... I had feelings akin to bereavement,

I think. . . . I felt terrible on every level: selfishly, professionally, in terms of my friends over there from both sides, Israelis and Palestinians, whom I wanted to be with. My drug had been taken away from me. For a period of five or six weeks I could not even bring myself to watch the news. I remember where I was when I finally made my decision to take up the BBC offer of the morning show. I was making a documentary about Jesus. We were filming in Petra, Jordan, and I was thinking about the new job, thinking and thinking. I had worked for the BBC for seventeen years and I didn't want to be just a one-trick guy, I suppose. Well, when I finally called them and said I was going to do it, I put the phone down and burst into tears. I could not bear it. . . . I thought, What have I done?"

Bowen's choice of language is noteworthy. He uses the same descriptors employed by substance abusers to depict their highs and periods of abstinence: exhilaration, brighter colors, my drug had been taken away from me, withdrawal symptoms. Once hooked on a drug, addicts may require escalating doses to achieve the same effect, a phenomenon termed tolerance. The analogy is once again striking in what Don McCullin had to say about his need for war. "I used to be a war-a-year man, but now that is not enough. I need two a year now. When it gets to be three or four, then I'll start to be worried." And Chris Dobson of the *Daily Mail* seals the association: "When I'm actually taking part in an action, it's always as though I'm three martinis up. I'm in another, a higher, gear and it's marvelous."

Comments such as these resonate with those of a cameraman I interviewed, whose behavior on occasion introduced a novel twist to the repertoire of sensation-seeking experiences. "There's nothing like getting shot at or shelled," he told me. "It's very exciting. Very frightening, very terrifying, but there is an awful lot of adrenaline running around. And adrenaline, as you probably know, is a very powerful drug. You live life with a much greater intensity. I remember having the experience, for example, of making love to a woman while being shelled. That's very intense. They're trying to extinguish life and you're trying, in theory, to create it. That's very strange. Everything would be that much more intense."

———

This drive for intensity, this need for new experiences, has been well documented in the behavioral science literature. Pivotal work has been done by Marvin Zuckerman and colleagues at the University of Delaware, who in the early 1960s began developing a rating scale to measure what they termed sensation-seeking behavior.* They defined this as the search for varied, novel and intense sensations and experiences, and the willingness to take physical, social, legal and financial risks to get them. Over a number of decades various forms of the scale were developed and refined, and in the process four cardinal features of sensation-seeking behavior were identified: thrill and adventure seeking, experience seeking, disinhibition and boredom susceptibility. Although in certain persons these four factors may coexist, the data from field studies suggested independent properties for each subscale.

The Sensation-Seeking Scale (SSS) has been widely used by investigators searching for a better understanding of this aspect of human behavior. Some demographic trends have been identified,

---

* Some war journalists take exception to terms such as this. James Nachtwey is one who peremptorily dismisses them as inaccurate. "I would reject the term 'novelty seeker.' That is definitely not the way I would describe myself or my colleagues. I think that I'm someone who did not want to lead a conventional life, but it wasn't novelty I was seeking, it was experience. Seeking some meaning in life, not novelty. I just think that it's not the right way of looking at it." While I am sensitive to the concerns of Nachtwey and those who share his opinion, I do not believe that words like "sensation," "novelty" and "adventure" diminish in any way the motives of journalists who may see themselves as visual historians or the voice of the oppressed. By using them I am simply tapping into terminology that is well established in the behavioral sciences and that comes without judgmental labels. No matter the semantics, to shy away from an impressive body of research because of a reluctance to offend does any discussion of motivation a disservice.

and they relate to the profile of war journalists. For example, data from the general population have consistently shown that men have higher scores than women. This helps explain my finding that three-quarters of all war journalists are male. There is also a clear relationship between SSS scores and age, although here the association is largely inverse. SSS scores start rising between nine and fourteen years of age (around puberty), peak in late adolescence and the early twenties and thereafter decline steadily. Bringing this observation back to my data, the match is again readily apparent. The mean age of my sample of 140 war journalists was the late thirties, with only 7 percent of active war journalists over fifty years of age.

A third demographic variable that deserves closer scrutiny is marital status. We've seen that under 45 percent of war journalists are married, which compares with a figure of greater than 80 percent in the age-matched general population. Here it is relevant to note that Zuckerman and colleagues found an association between high SSS scores and divorce, in both genders, but the etiological implications are unclear. Do high SSS scores lead to divorce, or does the breakup of a marriage lead to high SSS scores by forcing divorcés to adopt a more sensation-seeking lifestyle? Zuckerman's data do not let him answer the question, but in war journalists, where the case for sensation seeking pre-divorce is irrefutable, it is tempting to suggest that it is this very type of behavior that leads to marriages unraveling.

But although it is informative to extrapolate findings from the SSS data to my data and observe the close mesh, the fact that war journalists, like most sensation seekers, are predominantly young, male, single (or divorced) tells us nothing about why this should be so. To explore etiology, we need to look elsewhere, at heredity and neurophysiology in particular, for there is compelling evidence that journalists are genetically and biologically primed to pursue their particular type of work.

Studies of identical and fraternal twins have proved that well over 50 percent of the sensation-seeking trait is heritable, a figure that puts it at the upper end of the heritability range for most personality traits. But while these genetic findings are compelling, they cannot stand alone. Other factors such as environmental influences and error in measuring the sensation-seeking trait must be considered too. Yet even in a study of identical twins reared apart, the heritability rate for sensation-seeking behavior was 59 percent, powerful evidence that shared family environment does not necessarily have an impact on this particular personality trait.

Genes, however, do not directly control behavior. Rather, they determine an individual's neurophysiological makeup, and it is at this level that a few key neurotransmitters and hormones modulate novelty-driven behavior. Neurotransmitters are chemical messengers that carry information from one nerve (neuron) in the brain to another. Neurotransmission underlies every aspect of behavior, from gross movement to the subtlest thought. Hormones, in turn, are chemical messengers produced by a tissue or an organ. Unlike neurotransmitters, they travel in the bloodstream to exert effects on other tissues or organs, in the process also modifying behavior.

When war journalists speak of getting their adrenaline surge in combat zones, they are identifying one neurotransmitter that in popular imagination is the archetypal behavioral stimulant. Adrenaline (also called epinephrine) is an important agent released by the adrenal medulla in response to stress; it speeds up the heart rate, increasing the rate of breathing and inducing sweating, among other familiar reactions. But it is not the neurotransmitter that controls sensation-seeking behavior. That role falls to a distant relative, two steps removed, called dopamine.

The brain manufactures dopamine from an amino acid, tyrosine, found in dietary protein. Tyrosine is converted to a chemical L-dopa, a precursor to dopamine, which in turn is converted to noradrenaline by the enzyme dopamine-B-hydroxylase. Noradrenaline may then be transformed into adrenaline. Dopamine may also be broken down by the enzyme monoamine oxidase (MAO). With this basic knowledge we can see that dopamine, once formed, can be depleted by two routes, namely degradation via MAO or conversion to noradrenaline. And it is the influence of the MAO enzyme that has provided the most convincing evidence linking the seemingly disparate clinical, demographic, genetic and biochemical correlates of risk-taking behavior.

MAO, which is under tight genetic control, exists in two forms, A and B, and it is the latter that is active in the brain, where it breaks down dopamine. While it is not possible to directly measure brain MAO, an analogous form in blood platelets is quantifiable simply by taking a sample of blood. Many studies have explored the relationship between sensation-seeking behavior as measured by Zuckerman's scale (SSS) and levels of MAO, and the consensus is that high SSS scores are associated with low MAO levels. This inverse relationship has been consistently noted for both sexes. The inference is that low levels of MAO lead to high levels of dopamine, and that in turn manifests as pronounced sensation-seeking behavior. The converse is also true. MAO levels are higher in women and increase with age, which once again helps explain the war journalists' demographic profile.

––––––––––

The need for new sensations is only one possible motivating factor. The journalists who spoke to me all offered theories of personal motivation, of which the buzz of war was but a part. The photographer Gary Knight's perception is that a multiplicity of factors is to be found among his colleagues. "The Kosovo conflict is a very good example," he told me. "You would have a group of people working there who I would say were very, very, very finely tuned in to the political issues involved [in] what was at stake and in some way were addressing these issues. That is a very small number of people. Then you would have a really large number of people who were just there because CNN or the BBC sent them there and maybe the correspondent is driven by the same motives found in the small clique I have just mentioned, but the crew are there just because they are the crew. That is the largest group of news people who just happen to find themselves there. Maybe they have some experience in that area, but that's it. I am not being derogatory when I say this. They are not people for whom this life is a mission—for this group, it is a job, no more than that. Then you have a smaller number who are war junkies and completely get off on the adrenaline flying around. And then you have people within all those groups who have that as well. But the pure adrenaline junkies—and certainly there are a number of them—don't care what they are doing, who they are photographing. They don't give a shit about people being killed, about the trauma, they just care about the adventure. They are usually the guys you find walking over the mountains looking for the guerrilla groups, like I did when I was young."

Like Knight, all veteran war journalists I interviewed regarded these thrill seekers with contempt, even while many acknowledged that they too were galvanized by danger and threat. What in their minds distinguishes them from the self-serving, heedless adrenaline junkie is that they care passionately about those imperiled by conflict, the traumatized, dispossessed, bereaved victims that war spews forth with such disregard. "This life is a mission" is the credo by which Knight and his colleagues live and without which they too would be reduced to what the London *Times* correspondent Janine di Giovanni calls "the whackos, the adrenaline freaks, working for weird magazines like *Soldier of Fortune*, wearing khakis or soldier stuff and getting really excited by it all."

It is not just a sense of moral responsibility that keeps the war journalists aloof from the thrill-seeking buccaneer types. It is also a sense of personal preservation. There are dangers enough in war zones without getting too close to those whose actions are swashbuckling and irresponsible. Veteran war journalists have accumulated a considerable knowledge of survival techniques over the course of a decade or more working in zones of conflict, learned behaviors that contribute in no small measure to their longevity. The adventurer masquerading as a war journalist knows little, if any, of this. Prey to impulsivity, imbued with narcissism and with a penchant for daredevil antics, they are attracted to trouble like moths to a flame. In turn, they can quickly bring trouble down on their own heads. The case of Ken Hechtman illustrates the point.

"Kidnapped Journalist a Rookie with a Reckless Past: Once Stole Lab Uranium" ran a headline in Toronto's *National Post* newspaper at the height of the American-led war on the Taliban regime in Afghanistan. Described by an acquaintance as a "freelance everything, a jack of all trades," the thirty-three-year-old Hechtman decided just prior to the commencement of American bombing to become a journalist. Paying his own way to Pakistan, he crossed the border into Afghanistan, where he was quickly arrested by the Taliban, prompting efforts by Reporters without Borders and the Canadian government to procure his release. While he was in captivity some colorful episodes in Hechtman's past came to light. As a student in New York, he had stolen a small quantity of uranium from an unlocked physics laboratory "because it seemed like a neat thing to have," and he wanted to do "neat things with chemicals, simple experiments, minor pyrotechnics, that sort of thing." The deans, who placed Hechtman on disciplinary probation and ordered him out of student residence, also found him guilty of stealing a bathroom door and writing graffiti on a volunteer ambulance, among other offenses.

While Hechtman may have been looking for trouble, some journalists are in thrall to wanderlust, a hankering for distant, exotic lands that often takes root in childhood. Peter Arnett gives voice to this beautifully. He became known to millions of viewers as the Associated Press journalist who remained behind in Saigon in 1975, following the American pullout. More than a decade later, this time as the CNN man in Baghdad, he again stayed on while most of the networks left, and reported the dramatic opening shots of the 1991 Gulf War. In his memoir, *Live from the Battlefield*, he recalls a childhood growing up in Bluff, a small fishing town at the bottom end of New Zealand's South Island. "I was thrilled that it was home to the southernmost lamppost in the world, so certified by a sign at Stirling Point, where the waters of the Pacific Ocean and Tasman Sea met, crashing against the worn-smooth rocks. Nailed to the lamppost were distance and directional signs to the rest of the world painted in black on yellow wood: London, 12,608; New York, 10,005; Hamburg, 12,198; Tokyo, 6,389. Those signs mesmerized me as the Pied Piper bewitched the children of Hamelin. I would follow those signs and my dreams to the far reaches of the world."

Jeremy Bowen also retains this strong childhood memory: "I always wanted to be a foreign correspondent, even before I knew what it was," he told me. "I remember as a kid in school, when they went around the class and said what do you want to be, people would say astronaut, footballer, and I would say foreign correspondent. They would say what is a foreign correspondent and I didn't honestly know, but I had this vision of a newspaperman in a white suit with a fan going in the roof."

Several of the interviewees told of similar recollections, some no more than a fleeting, albeit never forgotten, memory. As a youngster, the photographer Santiago Lyon remembers walking in Ireland with his father and coming across a political demonstration. "There were a couple of photographers running around, and my father said, 'Wow, look at those guys. Do you want to be like one of them, wearing a leather jacket and traveling the world?' And I thought, That sounds all right." Janine di Giovanni knew as a child that she "never wanted to marry a doctor and play tennis. I wanted to be in the middle of the world." Fergal Keane recalled "just escaping into books about foreign places, far away places, fantasyland."

In the case of one war journalist, wanderlust combined with family discord, magnifying the impetus to seek out foreign wars.

"My father had a regular job working nine to five, and until a certain point in my life, I thought everybody did that. Then I saw a book by a photographer on the Vietnam War, and I bought it with my pocket money. When I read it I didn't understand how the book had come about. The interaction between the storytelling and the author didn't connect, and I couldn't understand how this person had gone off to this fantastic place and done this work. Yet it had to be a job, so there had to be things out there other than working nine to five. It was an adventurous, romantic notion. My parents divorced and I was fed up at home. I was frustrated. I wanted to be a photojournalist ever since I read that book at fourteen. I wanted even more to escape my home at seventeen, when my parents' acrimonious divorce reached a peak. For me, becoming what was in that book on Vietnam was a form of adventure and self-exploration. It was also a form of escapism, and I guess it was a form of punishment for my parents. I think it was many things."

Being smitten in youth with a desire for adventure and travel does not by itself translate into a career as a war journalist. But for some it does furnish one piece in a complex multidimensional puzzle, linked as travel, war and journalism are by unpredictability and risk. One of the great latter-day adventurers, the late Bruce Chatwin, addresses this very point in a collection of essays, *Anatomy of Restlessness*. "Travel must be adventurous," he writes. "The bumps are vital. They keep the adrenaline pumping around. . . . We all have adrenaline. We cannot drain it from our system or pray it will evaporate. Deprived of danger we invent artificial enemies, psychosomatic illnesses, tax-collectors and worst of all, ourselves, if we are left alone in the single room. Adrenaline is our travel allowance. We might just as well use it up in a harmless way."

Interspersed among Chatwin's essays on travels to well-worn byways in France and Italy are his memories of expeditions to Timbuctoo and Patagonia, and references to Bedouins and the Bushmen of the Kalahari. Chatwin, quoting from Robert Burton's seventeenth-century *Anatomy of Melancholy*, asserts that movement is the best cure for melancholy. It is no coincidence that the title of his essay collection paraphrases Burton's. The one's restlessness and the other's melancholia are intricately fused, sharing an anatomical substrate rendered either functional or dysfunctional by opportunity and the concentrations of pivotal neurotransmitters coursing through their central nervous systems. Burton yearned to travel, but circumstances thwarted his desire. Here Chatwin was more fortunate, and so their names became forever linked with melancholy and adventure respectively. Yet their shared insights, three centuries apart, highlight the biological drives underpinning motivation. For Chatwin, travel into the hinterland of Mali in search of Timbuctoo, navigating the Sahel and blistering heat of Saharan Africa, was not without risk, for he writes, "It has been claiming European victims and luring many to their deaths, since it first appeared on a Catalan map of the fourteenth century." This evocative city got his adrenaline going, spurred him on to new experiences and wondrous sights that in turn stimulated an outpouring of remarkable prose. Sated, he returned home, his self-professed *horreur du domicile* in temporary abeyance, grateful for a place where depleted resources could be replenished before restlessness again sent him on his way.

What sufficed for Chatwin, however, in terms of risk and novel experience is unlikely to satisfy the biological and psychological makeup of many war journalists. For them travel probably does little more than tickle abundant, dormant reserves of neurotransmitters but by itself is hardly likely to send levels ratcheting upward as an impetus to action. The inveterate traveler and war journalist may therefore share certain character attributes, but they do so differentially. For many war journalists, particularly when young and starting out on their careers, it is not just the risk of novelty that drives them but also the risk of danger. And because the latter is for obvious reasons the more intense experience, it often becomes the defining one. Placing your life on the line by venturing into the front lines of conflict zones cannot be surpassed.

Or can it? If getting mortared, bombed and shot at gives extreme risk takers that sought-after buzz, what do the perpetrators of violence experience? What emotions are they prey to as they inflict destruction on others? This question is not applicable to war journalists—for they are not combatants—but it is relevant when addressing the addictive qualities of violence. Evidence here suggests that, for some, the taking of life, given legitimacy in warfare, can prove an extraordinarily satisfying experience. Joanna Bourke's *An Intimate History of Killing* provides good evidence of this. She quotes the thoughts of one Capt. Julian Henry Frances Grenfell, a British First World War combatant responsible for sniping and killing a number of Germans over the course of many months, actions that in part earned him a Distinguished Service Order. "It is all the most wonderful fun; better fun than one could ever imagine. I hope it goes on a nice long time; but pigsticking will be the only tolerable pursuit after this one or one will die of sheer ennui." For Grenfell, life without license to kill man (preferably) or beast (second best), would be intolerably boring, yet despite the callousness of these remarks, there is no other evidence indicating he was some raging psychopath, devoid of the vestiges of compassion. At times he admitted to feeling "terribly ashamed" and regarded his enemy as "poor, dead Huns." Captain Grenfell, in the unabashed honesty of his writings, reveals himself to be an intense sensation seeker, who would have difficulty assuaging his desires even within the shifted spectrum of behavior followed by war journalists. War provided the outlet for this extreme drive, just as it unmasks similar traits in individuals who delight in its dark pleasures.

The examples given thus far clearly show that risk-taking behavior lies along a continuum. At the sedate end are found those persons who hold down the nine-to-five job, varying little in their daily routine. Shift the gauge away from this secure zone of predictability, and you start to encounter those whose behavior introduces a greater degree of uncertainty into their lives. Where you actually cross the threshold of what determines an adventurous life is arbitrary and subjective, but few would quibble that by the time you encounter a Bruce Chatwin, risk, adventure and novelty are well-ensconced lifestyle attributes. Shift the gauge further upward and you meet the war journalist, encamped a little below the summit of extreme risk-taking behavior occupied by the inveterate adrenaline junkie, whose life is governed largely by that perpetual search for the ultimate thrill.

———

Biological reductionism thus goes some way toward explaining why certain people choose war journalism as a profession and are prepared to take considerable risks over the course of a couple of decades to pursue it. However, genes and biochemistry alone cannot furnish the complete picture. We also need to look anew at environmental influences, heterogeneous rather than shared, as the twins-reared-apart data remind us. Here the search is no longer empirically focused, but it may help explain why some people choose a career as a war journalist as opposed to one as a policeman or extreme athlete, to give but two examples of high-risk occupations.

Notwithstanding the miscellaneous nature of this search, some discernible threads begin to emerge. Anthony Loyd, in his memoir of wars in Bosnia and Chechnya, has disclosed details of his family's military background. Loyd's father was a military man, and he had a poor relationship with him, a situation common to other war journalists. Of the twenty-two male war journalists I interviewed, five had fathers in the military or police, and without exception all harbored unfilial feelings ranging from indifference to loathing at some point in their relationships. For some, rapprochement came with age, while for others antipathy endured. In all but one case the son joined the military as a way of invoking or redeeming a father's affection and esteem. The depth of the relationship malaise, however, defied such cosmetic remedying, and the son remained emotionally bereft of a father but now with the added difficulty of finding himself adrift in an institution with tightly defined rules and regulations, intolerant of individuality and punitive toward dissent.

Stifled by the rigidity of army life, yet captive to early family influences that had steered them in that direction, these men resigned from the military and gravitated toward zones of conflict, where something as simple as a camera or notepad gained them entry. Here they very quickly realized they had found their true calling, ready access to war largely on their own terms and an opportunity to unleash a creativity they hadn't known they possessed. The work not only forced them to confront danger, as their fathers had done, but stimulated them to create remarkable images, in word and print, of remarkable events. In the process they received the respect and accolades of news agencies perennially on the lookout for talented youngsters prepared to risk war and bring back a good story. The prestigious awards that soon followed were powerful affirmations of their newfound worth and confidence. They were finally able to confront their absentee military fathers, either consciously or unconsciously, with the fact that they too had seen war, survived its horrors and made something positive of the experience.

———

Zones of conflict, with their loosely defined physical and personal boundaries, are attractive places for some people who are searching not only for meaning in life but also for personal identity. One photojournalist saw it as "a form of escapism, an adventure, where you can create your own persona. You can reinvent yourself. The job comes with all kinds of preconceptions as far as people on the outside world are concerned, something perhaps heroic about it, or romantic, that you can hide behind if you want to. It is a great place to disappear into and experience some very extreme sensations and punish people, find new people, punish yourself."

Time and again, my interviews unearthed evidence of family discord and a troubled upbringing. These journalists did not need cajoling to share their intimate recollections with me. Just the contrary. No sooner had I asked why they had chosen this career than they launched into emotional recollections of their childhoods and what dysfunctional parents they had had. They talked of role models who couldn't sustain a marriage and were often absent, drunk, verbally abusive and indifferent to the havoc they were bringing down on their children's heads. Many of these journalists shared the conviction that their painful, lonely and at times violent childhoods had been powerful, unconscious factors influencing career choice. This insight, however, invariably arrived late. It was only when they were well entrenched in their careers that they made any connection between their past and present lives. Such was the case for one well-known correspondent who, early in my study, when journalists were first being approached to take part, shared with me his insights on motivation. "I know that for a long time I tended to see the distress caused by my war experience in isolation, i.e., they were the direct consequences of witnessing traumatic events," he wrote. "It took some time for me to begin to look at the inner turmoil that propelled me toward war zones. They were comfortable, they were 'home,' a replay of the tension and fear with which I had grown up. War reporting allows you to remain in that place, to avoid the pain that comes with trying to accept yourself and your past. So many of the colleagues I met in war zones were the children of fractured or unhappy homes. No wonder we recognized each other, felt good together. And what value did we place on the sweetness of our own lives when we willingly, almost joyously, risked them every day?"

Only after seeking and receiving psychotherapy was this man able to draw an analogy between the family battles of his youth and the later conflict he would witness as a war journalist. "It was what I was used to. I grew up in it, you know, but I didn't understand this at the time. There was no way I could have understood this as a child, but I was reading something recently and it just jumped off the bloody page at me. It is possible to have post-traumatic stress disorder from your childhood. I grew up in a war zone. It was just madness. My father would break furniture and all the stuff that goes with that. I learned at a very early age these kinds of coping strategies, and this could explain why I now believe passionately in bearing witness to war, which is not unrelated to my sense as a kid that nobody bloody well heard me. Nobody ever heard."

A photojournalist, whose career before she took up a camera perhaps allowed for a quicker and more penetrating insight, sent me this e-mail comment from a distant, all-but-forgotten hellhole: "I worked as a psychiatric social worker prior to becoming a journalist and have always analyzed our little clan with a lot of interest. I think we are all rather self-destructive." These comments interleave with those of the print journalist Emma Daly. When we met for an interview in Madrid, she was pregnant and had taken a break from war reporting. Her memories of the war in Bosnia remained vivid, including one particular set of exchanges with colleagues. "It was one night, after dinner at the Holiday Inn, where we were all staying in 1994. Because of the shelling and sniping we couldn't go anywhere or do anything. We were sitting around this big table, and there were about fifteen of us present, and we took turns speaking about our childhoods. One of the female journalists was fifteen years old when her mother died, and her father did not want to set up home for her or her sister, so they were sent away to boarding school and would spend the holidays with different sets of relatives. Then there was another journalist whose father was this big-shot Hollywood agent who ran out on him and his mother, and their lifestyle changed from a big opulent mansion in Hollywood to living in a car. They were left destitute, and he did not see his father again until he was eighteen years old. And so it went on. When one of the journalists blurted out, 'My brother killed himself,' everybody burst out laughing because it was like some pathetic movie script, with the confessions getting more and more ridiculous. As everyone went around the table it just got sadder and sadder and more dramatic. There was only one man who had had a normal childhood, and he was like, 'Gee guys, sorry, but my story is different.' Sarajevo was very much a place for black humor."

In my interviews, the theme of an unhappy childhood came with many variations. "You may wish to consider pre-war conditions that I am certain many journalists have" was one piece of advice given to me early. "It is one reason why many journalists are driven to cover wars. You may note, for example, that many hard-core war journalists have few, if any, photographs of family members or loved ones anywhere in their homes." I had no way of verifying this last claim, but it does disclose one insider's perspective of a highly defended profession, whose members are sometimes incapable of forming lasting attachments with family.

Some journalists went so far as to suggest that family malaise was virtually endemic. "In my profession, photojournalism, I would say eight out of ten of my colleagues have fairly dysfunctional backgrounds: a parent or both parents dead, divorced, stuff like that," one man told me. Six months later, in an interview on a different continent with another journalist, these observations were spontaneously repeated and the percentage endorsed. "There was a lot of instability in my life. I remember very clearly when my parents separated, and they didn't do it very well. It was a bit messy. I remember them fighting a lot. I remember being abandoned a lot, left alone a lot. I'm convinced it had something to do with the way things turned out. If you sit around a table of foreign correspondents or photographers or people who run around and do this business, I've found out that around 80 percent will have something similar, something screwed up. I think that initially, until you get that out of your system, and some people never do, that influences your later behavior."

Of the twenty-eight interviews I completed, a little more than 40 percent revealed a troubled childhood characterized by divorce or poor relationships between the nascent journalist and his parents. The most bizarre example of how distorted family relationships could become was offered by a cameraman whose parents were divorced when he was a toddler. He was never told this and always assumed his stepfather was his true dad. His mother, somewhat dissolute of habits, continued to lead a chaotic life, her two priorities being a good party and a ready supply of booze. Among the many men who frequently visited the home was someone introduced to the child as his uncle. Only as an adult did this cameraman learn that the man was really his biological father.

Informative as these anecdotes are, it is important to remember that recall is often subject to bias, the events of childhood potentially colored by troubled adult lives. Furthermore, divorce is common in the societies from which I drew my sample, and while a twenty-five-year follow-up study of children from broken marriages paints a disquieting picture of lives often emotionally unfulfilled, such outcomes are not invariable. This theory is also difficult to reconcile with the personal histories of those war journalists who come from loving, intact families, where relationships with parents are close and nurturing. These limitations aside, we can conclude that association clearly equals causality to some journalists, and their difficult childhoods are considered the root cause of an unsettled future spent wandering the globe in search of conflict.

———

Divorced parents; aloof, dysfunctional military fathers; troubled families; rudderless young men and women in search of identity and meaning and that missing family—if I have dwelled on these factors first and at length, it is because in my interviews with war journalists these were the issues raised most often and with the most spontaneity. However, there was a group of war journalists who experienced none of this domestic turmoil. Their largely middle-class family backgrounds were uncomplicated and happy.

What, then, is their motivation? Some, to be sure, were people we would regard as high sensation seekers, men and women with a drive for thrill and adventure. But others expressed a strong dislike for the bang-bang: these journalists were fearful of risk and apprehensive of the many threats that lurked in zones of conflict. What beguiled them was the drama of the events they were witness to. Time and again the war journalists, when asked about motivation, would respond, "I've been around history for the past ten years, and it's a privileged ringside seat too." Then they would smile somewhat sheepishly and apologize for the cliché. Yet bearing personal witness to the memorable events of history was only part of the story, as the more perceptive among them realized. What their status as war journalists offered was something equally heady: unheard-of access to the living rooms of citizens around the globe. It was through the imprint of their text and image that the great mass of humanity was kept informed.

The way war journalists rise to these challenges varies considerably. For some, war becomes a conduit to self-aggrandizement, stroking an ego that allows little space for competitors, be they fellow journalists or the victims of catastrophe. To others, it is simply a job, and while at times they marvel at the spectacle of it all, or are moved by it, it generally amounts to little more than a way to make a living. And then there is that small group, those Gary Knight characterized as being finely tuned to all the nuances of the conflict, who are not only alert to the broad political sweep of events, but whose antennae are able to detect, among the convulsions of a nation, those unforgettable individual cases of suffering and heroism that suffuse the events of war with such pity and poignancy.

Conscious of their responsibility in bearing witness, aware of the privilege their access afforded them, these war journalists have often invested their entire being, their physical strength, their emotional resources and their intellect in telling the story of war. To Janine di Giovanni, it became imperative to view personally what she wrote about. "What is this front-line stuff? What has happened in this battle? I feel you cannot write about it unless you see it. You just cannot write about it. I believe it is fundamentally dishonest to take information from other journalists and write about it. Things happen to you if you are in a country at war, and that gives you a precious insight into what the war is about. A lot of journalists covered the Chechnya story from Moscow. The average reader living in London would not know this and think the journalist was in the middle of a war. But they were not. They were sitting in a nice comfortable hotel."

Maggie O'Kane of the *Guardian* newspaper expounded on this theme; she told me that if war journalists want to write about war and the victims of war, they cannot turn their backs on these victims once the dangers start to mount. "I had this sense of mission in Baghdad. It was 1991 and the coalition was going to bomb the city. Fifteen of us decided to stay. I stayed because a colleague of mine said to me, 'There are very few times that we can actually be a bit useful and this is one of them.' In addition, I was too ashamed to leave. I was with a taxi driver, and we had been together for about ten or twelve days. He had ten children, and during the time he had brought me into his life. You know, I come in and his wife is cutting up the tablecloth to make gas masks. There was this kind of closeness and intimacy with him, and I felt ashamed to leave him and say I'm sorry, you're going to have the shit bombed out of you and I'm off. I've got a sense of responsibility, and when I said goodbye to him, as I did initially, I got out the car and felt my face go completely red in embarrassment. I recognized that as shame. So therefore I thought I had to stay, that it would prove useful, that we should be there. And the same thing happened in Bosnia, this sense that we the press had to be there. We have to stop this madness. That's why I do this job. Otherwise, why bother."

"How do you connect with what people are going through?" asked James Nachtwey, and his answer, quietly given, revealed a steely resolve. "Through your photographs, that's how. You have

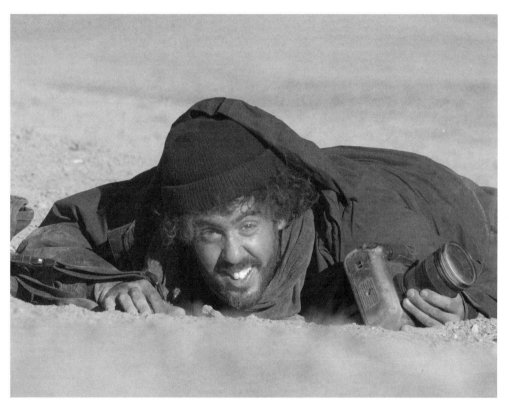

Photojournalist Ron Haviv of the photo agency VII dives for cover while under sniper fire from the Northern Alliance during the Taliban surrender of the village of Midan Shar near Kabul in 2001.

SCOTT PETERSON/GETTY

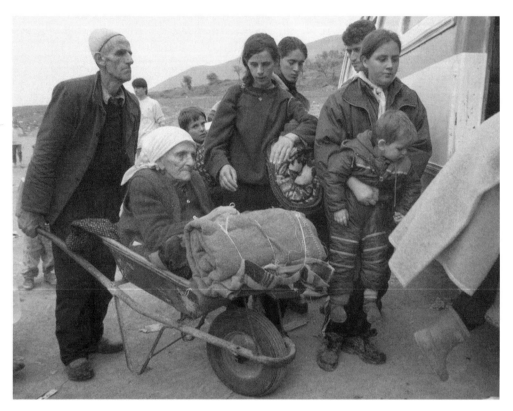

An elderly ethnic Albanian refugee woman waits in a wheelbarrow at the Kosovo border. More than 675,000 ethnic Albanians fled Kosovo after the NATO airstrikes began in March 1999. Many say they were forced out by roving bands of Serbs, and spoke of mass atrocities.

SANTIAGO LYON/AP

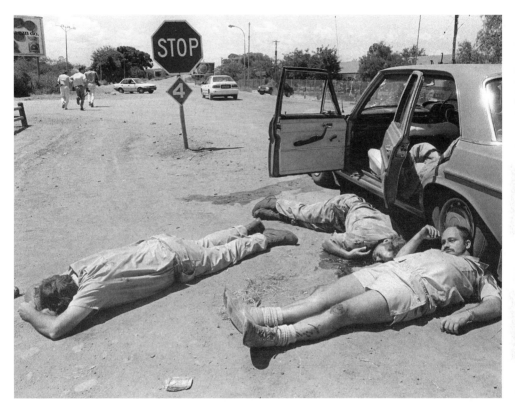

Journalists run from the scene of the roadside execution of members of the AWB, an extreme right Afrikaner movement, by a Bophuthatswana policeman. The summary killings came after an abortive AWB attempt to prop up the puppet apartheid regime in the homeland of Bophuthatswana in 1994.

GREG MARINOVICH

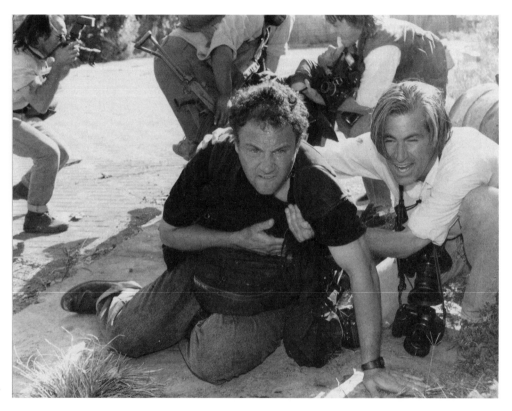

James Nachtwey (front right) assists a wounded Greg Marinovich, while in the background Joao Silva photographs Gary Bernard and an officer from the National Peacekeeping Force as they carry away the fatally wounded Ken Oosterbroek at Thokoza, South Africa, 1994.

JUDA NGWENYA

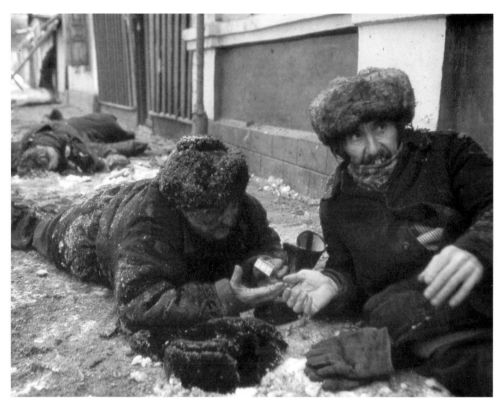

This image is from a sequence of photos of an artillery attack on civilians in Grozny. The two men in the foreground were injured (one lost both his legs). The only thing that Jon Jones, the photographer, was able to do for them was to offer cigarettes.

JON JONES

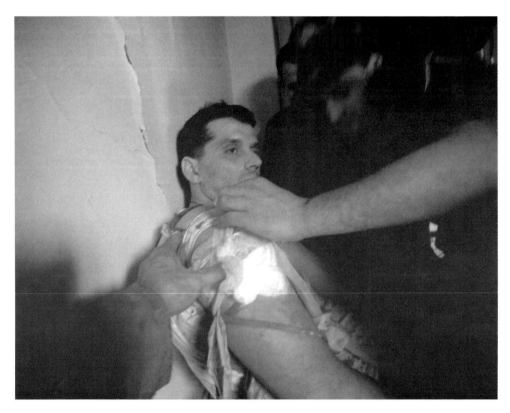

The injured soldier in this photo had been standing beside Jon Jones
when he was hit by sniper fire in Mostar. (Jones' arm appears on the left,
offering assistance.) He and others offered first-aid until they were able
to get the injured man out under the cover of fire.

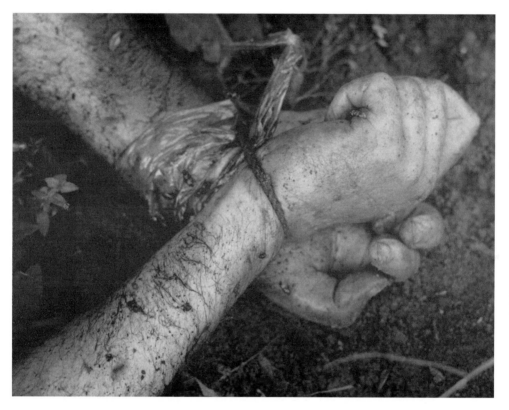

This man was executed by the side of a dirt track in Kosovo a few days after liberation by NATO forces.

GARY KNIGHT/VII

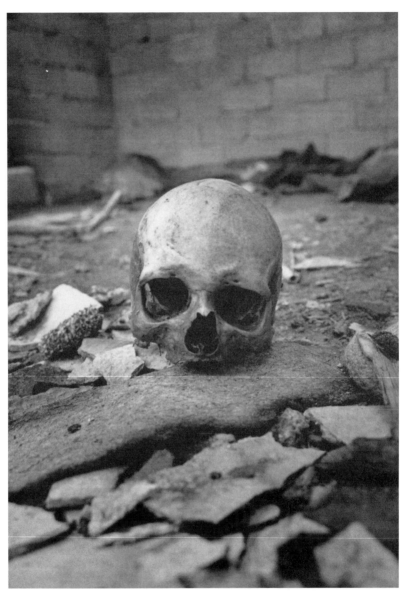

The skull and remains of a young woman who had been raped and murdered in an animal shed by the side of a road near Velika Krusha. Many
refugees who fled Kosovo during the NATO bombing recounted stories
of Serb soldiers taking young women from convoys of refugees.

to put yourself in the same space that they are in, and when you are in that same space, you experience the same risks. So you are sharing that with the people you are photographing. But it was never for the sake of taking a risk. It was risky because it was required to get the job done. And that's how I always felt about it and how I still feel about it. I'm still willing to take the risk to get the job done. That hasn't changed."

To be finely tuned to the issues at stake in a particular conflict while at the same time getting a buzz from the dangers involved are not necessarily incompatible. Indeed, it was my impression that the majority of committed career war journalists, those who had been working for a decade or more, combined both facets in varying ratios. However, it was only from the small ranks of the knowledge-able that I encountered those journalists who were the very antithesis of the thrill-and-adventure-seeking personality. Cognizant of the myriad dangers that zones of conflict presented, they waged a constant internal battle with their fears, misgivings and confidence when breaking news demanded they enter the front lines.

"One of the first times I felt myself to be in this position, of having to decide, was just before the Gulf War," recalled Allan Little. "There were maybe twenty of us. We were from different news organizations. We were suddenly granted visas and told to be ready by midnight the next day. So we had twenty-four hours to find the trucks, load them with food and water and petrol. It was a tense and horrible day. There were a few who just seemed excited by the whole thing. I was both excited and scared. It wasn't just the physical danger—the thought that this could get you killed. I think I was also frightened by the magnitude of the story. It was the biggest thing I'd been trusted with, and I didn't know whether I'd be up to it or just lost. I was convinced that I was surrounded by people much more sure of what they were doing than I was. So I was scared in several different ways.

"We had a big meeting a few hours before our departure. There were some American TV journalists who had visas and were having cold feet about going. We would have to make the journey up the same road that the Scud missile launchers firing at Israel were coming down, so vehicles on that road were being bombed by the allies. A couple of the Americans were arguing that we shouldn't go unless we got a guarantee from the Pentagon of safe passage. I thought, Well, this is just not going to happen. Forget it. You're not going to get a guarantee of safe passage from the Pentagon. I thought they were just looking for a way not to go. There was just no way to make this journey safe. They were trying to measure the risk, asking, How safe is this? And I thought, You're trying to measure the unmeasurable. You just have to make a judgment about it. You have to make a pact with your own feelings, make a deal with yourself. I hadn't said anything at this meeting. I was one of the youngest there and the least experienced in war zones. But I heard myself say, 'You're trying to measure the unmeasurable. It can't be done. You must just decide whether you want to do it or not. If you don't want to go nobody blames you. It's a personal decision.' And when I said that the meeting kind of wound up. I hadn't intended to close off the discussion, but afterward a couple of the more gung-ho reporters there—those who had no doubts at all that they wanted to go—came up and said, 'Good for you, you spoke for us all.' And I thought, Well, I didn't mean to speak for us all. If only you knew how stressed I am about whether to go!

"A bit later I bumped into a photographer I knew who was very anxious about the whole thing, and he said, 'Are you going?' I said yes, and he said, 'Why? Why?' And all I could come up with was 'Because if I don't I'll never forgive myself. I'll regret it all my life.'"

If there is no emotional high waiting alongside danger, if the resolve to confront the risks is not spurred by the buzz that comes with such actions, then the job presents a different set of challenges: making a pact with your own feelings, gaining mastery of fear (never truly accomplished), weighing your emotional reserves. War journalists who feel this way find their motivation primarily in two sources, their often fierce ambition and the content of the story.

Ambition, of course, is often just as prevalent in the overweening narcissist as it is in the more high-minded journalist. It's just that the war journalists who are leery of risk, who do not place themselves at the center of the story, have to access motivation in another way. Still, in the end, ambition is a common denominator linking virtually all in the profession. They know that the kudos earned on the front lines is a good way of gaining recognition and advancing up the ladder. They have all seen examples of a career becalmed because a colleague lacked the "right stuff."

Commitment to the story, the desire to bear witness and keep the world informed, the drive to expose a great moral outrage—these become the issues by which a subset of journalists define themselves. The magnitude of the story to be told counterbalances the anxiety felt in zones of conflict, pushing them yet again to go down that road, not knowing what hazards lie around the corner. One cynical voice within the profession, however, scoffed at the moral high-mindedness of some of his colleagues. "I think there is an altruistic motive," he told me, "but I also think that a lot of people are not being entirely honest with themselves. Because you know what the answer is that people want to hear? They want to hear that you do it for the idealism and to save the world. I think it takes a rare degree of courage to say, 'Well, I actually love this.' It takes self-awareness to see that you do it for other reasons as well. If I had met you ten years back I probably would have avoided you like the plague. But if you had persuaded me to sit down with you and talk, I would have angrily denied that I did this work for anything other than my mission to speak on behalf of the dispossessed. It's easier to do that."

Reflecting on this observation, I wondered whether this journalist was not being too harsh in his peer assessment, holding his colleagues to a higher set of values. Ambition, self-promotion, choosing an occupation because of its rewards while espousing altruistic motives—the same could be said for many professionals. The war journalists I asked to comment on motivation all looked back on many years' cumulative experience when formulating their answers. They spoke freely about the thrill of danger, their ambition, the challenges they found stimulating, their mission as messengers of war. Many stated openly and without reservation that they loved the work. Where they differed was in defining exactly what it was they loved. For some, the primary impetus was a need to tell a remarkable story, one whose meaning transcends conflicts of nationality, religion and culture, even as it embraces all of them. For a small clique of journalists, Bosnia in the last decade of the twentieth century was a case in point.

"Bosnia was many things for us," a senior BBC journalist explained to me. "I personally felt it was Europe going back to the past. I felt it was important to understand it and not shut it out. I felt some kind of responsibility as a citizen. I grew up in the twentieth century with fine declarations, in an atmosphere in which we all believed there would never be another Holocaust. We all believed that if it happened this time, the world wouldn't stand for it. . . . I was burning with indignation, and I saw a clear injustice. I saw my own country and most of the allies ignoring it. I felt tainted by that. I felt that I had some kind of responsibility to stand up. I couldn't bear the shame of it, and in the end that's why I stopped covering Bosnia. I couldn't bear it.

"The war tore apart a society that closely resembled my own as a European. You could see that what happened there wasn't uniquely Balkan or a Yugoslav phenomenon. It was European. It was something that marked European history, and it seemed to me that Europe was in some ways going back to its past, and I felt bound up in it, wrapped up in it. Bosnia drew us all in. Bosnia also represented clear choices, moral choices, choices about the kind of values you adhered to. At the time the Bosnian war was happening, all the Western governments except the United States, which was very much in the background at first, were saying, 'It's a Balkan thing, savages, they've been killing each other for centuries. What can you do—they're all as bad as each other.' Those of us who were there knew that wasn't true. We absolutely knew that was a lie those governments used to justify their own inaction. And because we knew that, it involves a kind of responsibility.

"There was a criminal elite running one side of the conflict. They chose to have war because it was the only way they could stay in power. They planned the ethnic cleansing, resourced it, funded it, executed it, drove it, believed in it. They believed in it ideologically, as much as they did it. They thought it was a good thing. The other side wanted multi-ethnicity, tolerance, human rights, membership in the European club. One side aspired to what was good about Europe, and the other side wanted some kind of ethno-fascist project, which was also drawing on a certain supposedly discredited European tradition. So you have two European traditions here in conflict with each other. And if you make them morally the same, you are morally compromising yourself. And it seemed to all of us who were there that there was some kind of moral responsibility. It was our Spain, in a way. We had a choice to make. We could go along with the rubbish, but it wasn't true.

"These are the reasons why I think you've really got just one war in you. I think you can only commit yourself in that way once in your life, only believe in it once. It's like virginity—you can't lose it twice. When the disillusionment has entered your soul, once you understand that you are not doing any good at all, you cannot commit yourself in that same way a second time. I don't think I've ever articulated this because I just took it for granted. I genuinely believed that in the world I grew up in and was part of, if such a gross injustice existed, all that had to happen was for it to be made clear. For it to be spelled out. You could summon the force of international righteousness and the injustice would be ended. It took me about four years to understand that this was a childish delusion, that you can't summon the force of moral indignation, because the freedom citizens are enjoying includes the freedom not to care.

That terrible disillusionment fixes itself, and that is why I think you can only do it once. We've all got just one in us."

This articulate voice speaks for other war journalists whose careers were also defined by events in Bosnia. And yet, even this man remembers being thrilled by the sound of gunshots going off near him in Bucharest early in his career. "That was the first time I heard a gun go off in anger," he told me. "It was great. I loved it and I was good at dealing with it and I'd found something that I could do well and I was being rewarded for it." Does such a reaction lessen his conviction or invalidate his moral argument? How can we reconcile the cogent, eloquent and passionate motivation espoused in Bosnia with a different reaction in Bucharest? As I got to know the profession better, I came to realize that there was no contradiction, no self-deception, that all the reasons applied in their own way, and that one of the most important variables that controls which motivating factor predominates at any one point in time was age. As one war photographer said to me, "The reasons I started doing this as a young man and the reasons I still do it are probably largely different. There has been a readjustment, although some core features remain immutable, such as I do it well and I am able to earn a living by it. I think I was foolish at times when I was younger, but I think that is just youth. Now I do this work because I am more empowered, I am a better photographer, a better storyteller and I have a better conscience, a better understanding of what is right, what is wrong, what is moral, what is ethical. I didn't know black from white when I was younger."

This evolution in motivation was common to that small group of "finely tuned" war journalists. Youthful impetuosity, that thirst for adventure spiced with risk, owes much to individual biochemistry and factors that modulate dopamine. War journalism offers an outlet to assuage that innate drive. Exposed to remarkable events, privy to suffering on a grand scale, moved by the plight of war's victims, some journalists begin to realize, with time, that their job is more than a series of exotic escapades. This emotional maturation includes a heightened sensitivity to those nameless people left dispossessed, powerless and grieving by war. In consort with this changing outlook, biochemical changes are occurring too; MAO levels are increasing and dopamine levels are declining, leading to a dwindling desire for those daredevil escapades that, in retrospect, evoke a shudder. It is not an all-or-nothing transformation, of course. Some frisson of excitement persists with time, just as an element of moral indignation was probably there to start off with. Over the course of a decade or two, the risk-morality ratio gets recalibrated.

For some journalists, neither risk nor morality is highly relevant—war journalism is simply a job. For others, the degree of recalibration will vary according to the individual. This model, which fits together widely disparate motivational factors, may help explain one journalist's assertion that he was good for one war only. In support of his theory, I have noticed there are other war journalists who also tend to define their careers by a single major conflict. These are frequently protracted civil wars that entice foreign military intervention. Thus, the past quarter century has seen the Vietnam generation, the Beirut generation and more recently, the Bosnian generation of war journalists. The long duration of conflict provides sufficient time for a motivational shift to occur, and given what a formative influence it has on the journalists' outlook, no subsequent conflict will ever again attain the same degree of intensity. Even for those journalists who do not follow this transformation, the simple passage of time, associated as it is with a fall-off in neurotransmitter levels, may mean that when peace wearily supervenes, their love for the bang-bang has peaked. Both groups will move on to other wars, where their skills honed in conflict together with aptitude will ensure the quality of their work. But some will always look back, either in bitterness or nostalgia, on that one all-embracing, career- and life-defining war.

It is understandable that, given the risks war journalists take, they should at times question their motives. This self-examination becomes particularly acute when their lives are directly threatened. When the immediate threat subsides, however, and survival emerges victorious yet again, the urge to question rapidly disappears from consciousness. Paradoxically, the intensity of the close call may be one of the factors that draws the journalist back into the zones of conflict. But the death of a colleague and especially age can have the greatest dampening effect on motivation. By the time journalists reach their forties, they are faced with new pressures: a need to settle down and have children, or the demands of a partner who, after a decade or more functioning largely as a single parent, delivers the ultimatum. And then there are the biochemical changes that occur with aging. We have already looked at the effects of an increase in MAO and fall-off in dopamine concentration. Alongside these chemical changes comes a physical slowing-down. War journalism is physically taxing. Walking up a mountainside in the heat of an African summer or the snow and ice of a Balkan winter is far easier for a young journalist than twenty years later, particularly when the intervening period has included generous quotas of alcohol and cigarettes. If they want to get out into the field, if they want to be seen on the front lines, gathering their own facts, journalists need to forsake their creature comforts. These privations were not lost on Evelyn Waugh during his brief stint as a foreign correspondent. Trapped for days on end with a large group of locals and a single lavatory among them, he complained somewhat bitterly to his editor back home that every time he went for a shit he vomited instead. Seventy years later the sanitation issue remains no less taxing. In an article entitled "One Toilet and the World's Press Wants It," Janine di Giovanni described conditions in Khoje Bahwudine in northern Afghanistan. "The place has virtually no infrastructure. Water comes from the river, carried by donkeys. Sleep is on the floor, if you are lucky. I have not slept three nights in the same place. Journalists were sleeping in hallways, sleeping outside the stinking hole that served as a toilet, sleeping on the concrete verandah. Confrontation began when the press corps woke up and began fighting for water and electricity. At one point one toilet was shared by everyone, but NBC bought the house temporarily and hung up a sign, This Room Is Property of NBC."

Such esprit de corps is easier to tolerate when young.

———

When plotting the reasons why war journalists choose such hazardous work, we can see there are few absolutes. This should not come as a surprise, for an explanation of the complexities of behavior demands a synthesis of many factors. A spectrum of traits, a continuum of responses, thresholds, ratios, probabilities—this is the language in which etiological theories of behavior are couched. Yet despite the imprecise nature of our understanding, we have many strands of evidence that shed light on why war journalists take this particular path in life. None of these factors—biochemical, environmental, political, moral—can stand alone, but when taken together they produce a coherent and persuasive argument. Devising a model to fit every possible permutation, however, treats all war journalists equally, whereas from a behavioral point of view, they differ in terms of interest. By focusing on that relatively small group whose creativity in zones of conflict has shaped our impressions of war, we can distill certain core truths in relation to motivation. That level of war journalism is seldom, if ever, achieved by those who regard their work as simply another job. When the primary motivating factor is the paycheck at the end of the month, imagination and ingenuity languish. That is not to decry these journalists' technical skill, but technique in the absence of passion usually leaves us unmoved. Similarly, the journalists driven solely by thrill-seeking behavior will seldom sustain a career. Dismissed by their colleagues as habitual adrenaline junkies, they may be good for only a quick war or two before they move on to other sources of titillation. Finally, we can also split off those journalists whose narcissism gets in the way of the story, for by positioning themselves center stage they deflect the spotlight away from combatants and victims. In doing so, they contaminate the news.

This leaves a group of journalists, few in number, whose mission is defined by their desire to go to the heart of a conflict and tell the story of those who wage war, those who are destroyed by it and those who rise above it. They get a buzz from the adventure. Satisfaction comes from a job well done. There is pride in the awards that follow. We simply note all this in passing, for these are universal responses and should not detract from what these journalists do. In the end, what moves them is ultimately what moves us as human beings: tragedy unlocking the grandeur of the human spirit. Each of the war journalists I spoke to lent credence to this with a series of remarkable anecdotes. From these I have selected one haunting image with which to close this chapter. The photojournalist Jon Jones, trapped atop the Caucasus with refugees. A family's worldly possessions in a car. In Jones's honor, the wife prepares a meal with what little she has. A white tablecloth is found and spread across the car's hood. The father rummages among the boxes. He unearths a bottle of champagne. He had been saving it for the birth of his son. But the journalist has braved grave dangers to tell their story. His courage must be saluted.

4

DEATH, DEPRESSION, DRINK AND DRUGS

As you empty the bottles you refill them with your soul.

— GÉRARD DE NERVAL

The war against the Taliban in Afghanistan provides bleak evidence of the high mortality rate that comes with telling war's story. In just over one week, eight journalists were killed. Among them was Julio Fuentes, ranked as one of the half-dozen most experienced war journalists of his generation by the *Guardian*'s John Hooper. There is nothing new in war journalists' dying violent deaths, but even for this hardy profession, the degree of carnage in Afghanistan was unusual. Soon after I began my study, Kurt Schork and Miguel Gil Moreno were killed. Eighteen months later, the murder of Julio Fuentes triggered the same intense mix of sadness and bewilderment. "I still cannot believe Julio Fuentes is dead, even after seeing the crematorium curtains close silently before his coffin," grieved his friend and fellow war journalist Emma Daly in her *Observer* column. What made these particular deaths so unsettling for journalists, apart from the pain of personal loss, was that they were yet another reminder that no combination of experience, skill, intelligence, compassion and caution can prevent some tragedies. In discussing the loss of a colleague and friend, Jerome Delay recalled, "When we were all at Miguel's funeral, we looked at each other and wondered who was going to be next." The answer was not long in coming. And as the doors of the crematorium swung closed behind Fuentes's coffin, the same thought was no doubt rekindled once more.

———

Bereavement can at times merge into clinically significant depression. Furthermore, one in two patients with PTSD, the quintessential trauma reaction, may also have an associated depression. For these reasons, I felt it was important for my study to include an assessment of journalists' mood. A widely used self-report questionnaire, the Beck Depression Inventory, was therefore given to all participants. This scale lists twenty-one symptoms of depression and assesses the severity of mood change by scoring the responses as minimal, mild, moderate or severe. When the results of the Beck scale for the 140 war journalists and the 107 non-war group were compared, the former were found to be significantly more depressed. A closer examination revealed that severe depression was uncommon in both groups of journalists, but more war journalists fell into the moderate category. Most of the domestic journalists had only minimal or mild depression scores. This difference was again statistically significant.

Of the twenty-one symptoms of the Beck Depression Inventory, those most often reported by the war group include: sadness; past failure; loss of pleasure; guilty feelings; self-criticalness; suicidal thoughts or wishes; crying; loss of interest; indecisiveness; change in sleep patterns; irritability; and loss of interest in sex. Pessimism, agitation and change in appetite were also reported, though less frequently. There was no one symptom that was more prominent among domestic journalists. The list demonstrates the extent to which sufferers of depression experience symptoms other than sadness, and it helps explain why depression can be such a debilitating disease. Yet the Beck self-report scale, while informative, cannot be used to generate a clinical diagnosis. For that, a structured interview is required. This was completed on the random sample of twenty-eight war journalists, and it revealed a lifetime prevalence of major depression approaching 22 percent.* The equivalent figure for clinically meaningful major depression in the United States is approximately 5 percent, which corresponded to the level noted among the domestic journalists.

Although the association between depression and loss is well documented in the psychiatric literature, the relationship takes on special meaning when it comes to war journalists. No experienced member of the profession has been spared the violent death of a colleague. Focusing therefore on a more discrete group—namely, those who have lost a close working partner, someone with whom they have braved the front lines and endured many shared dangers —becomes more informative. "In this business, there's a kind of forced closeness because of what you do," explained Greg Marinovich, the South African stills photographer, describing his working relationships. The intensity of this shared existence forges strong bonds of friendship that in some cases supersede ties to family. Anthony Loyd, for example, was estranged from his father but wears a locket containing some of Kurt Schork's ashes.

For some journalists, when death takes a colleague the sense of loss is not only profound but, depending on circumstance, often stoked by guilt. What befell Allan Little during his time as one of the BBC's Balkan correspondents is one such example.

"Bosnia was really tough in '92," he told me. "I was absolutely committed to the story. I believed in the importance of being there. It was under my skin. In October I was in central Bosnia. There was a sudden huge refugee exodus. I called my office and said,

---

* One journalist's diagnosis of major depression predated his work in war zones.

'You should see this—it's huge. You must send me a cameraman.' Well, they did send me someone—a friend of mine—we'd worked together in Bosnia and in Croatia the previous year. He drove up from the coast, we spent the day filming together and then spent the night sleeping on the floor of someone's apartment. The next day we swapped cars—I took his little soft-skinned hire car and gave him the armored Land Rover. I headed back to the coast to a place where I could edit and transmit the report. He waited in central Bosnia and was due to be joined by another correspondent the next day. Half an hour after I left him he was killed. A Serb gunner fired an armor-piercing anti-aircraft round horizontally through the cab of his car.

"I fell apart after that. I thought it was my fault. I couldn't imagine ever 'getting over' this. I felt guilty just for being alive. I remember the moment I was told he'd been killed, and I simply didn't believe it. I said, 'No—you're wrong. I've just seen him. He's alive. You're mistaken.' I argued with the man who broke the news to me. The next day we got up at six and drove back into Bosnia to collect his body. We took a hearse. I think the reality of what had happened hit on the way back, when we'd picked up the body. I think I wanted to swap places with him. I knew that if, at that moment, some divine authority had come down and said, 'You have a choice, it could be him or you,' I would have said, 'Okay, me.' I felt totally wretched about being alive."

Writing in the *Evening Standard* eight years later, Little noted, "I became withdrawn and moody. I couldn't sleep without nightmares. I started to fear the night. I drank too much, which made everything worse. I even grew paranoid and began to imagine that people were talking about me. I didn't realize any of this at the time, but some of my friends thought I was going mad and had become dangerously obsessed."

Like most of the journalists I interviewed, Little was difficult to pin down. When we finally met at a café in Johannesburg, we had only an hour to chat before he was off to catch a plane back to London en route to Yugoslavia. Events in the Balkans were once again moving quickly, but for a change they appeared headed in a positive direction. Thousands of demonstrators had taken to the streets of Belgrade, and Slobodan Milosevic was about to be toppled. During the interview Little was by turns happy and sad, excited about the imminent fall of the Yugoslav dictator and somber as he recalled the death of his cameraman. "In the weeks that followed I began to feel that any sort of enjoyment of life from now on was unthinkable. I thought it would be impossible ever to laugh again, ever to dance or just have a happy time or enjoy myself. I thought it would be a betrayal. I was also very angry. I wanted to kill the person who had done it. I wanted to go to the gun position, because I knew exactly where the thing had been fired from, and I really did want to go to that place and kill the guy who had done it."

Little's symptoms of loss of pleasure and guilt are typical of the grieving process. Some mourners may experience more unusual symptoms, such as a temporary disturbance in their perception. This may include hearing the voice or catching a fleeting glimpse of the deceased. These "micro" hallucinations are extremely brief, lasting only a few seconds before reality intervenes. They also occur almost exclusively during the acute period of grief, which by definition should not last longer than two months. The persistence of these altered perceptions beyond this period suggests bereavement merging with a more ominous depression.

Some journalists who have lost close colleagues describe experiences like these. In one case, the hallucinations persisted for two years. This journalist, who had survived a particularly harrowing ordeal in the Middle East, would see a dead colleague in crowds or walking down the street toward him. He would also have vivid dreams in which his friend featured prominently. What troubled him about the dreams was their lifelike intensity: many of the dead man's idiosyncrasies, mannerisms, foibles—in short, all the personality characteristics that made him such a distinctive individual— were perfectly re-enacted. At times the hallucinations were so authentic that the journalist came to doubt whether his colleague had indeed been killed. These re-enactments, whether during consciousness or sleep, triggered considerable guilt and depression. For relief he turned increasingly to alcohol and cocaine, both of which can interfere with sleep architecture, heightening the floridness of the already altered perceptions.

Jeremy Bowen was covering a story in the Middle East when he too lost a close colleague and friend, although in his case the death was witnessed firsthand. It was 2000 and Israel was in the processing of withdrawing its army from southern Lebanon. Bowen and his longtime Lebanese driver, Abed Takkoush, were following the progress of disengagement. Their car stopped in an area they considered safe, and Bowen got out of the vehicle and moved off to a vantage point. Then a shell hit the car.

"I spun around because I had my back to it, and there was this huge fireball. I didn't realize it was the car to start with, then I realized it was. And at that moment I saw him lurching out of the driver's window and he was just on fire. He slumped on the road. What went through my head was first to go up and see if I could help him, but my second thought was not to go, it would be horrible, he would be in a terrible state and would probably be dead. The third thought was the most sensible one. I had done a combat first-aid course with the BBC, and they said the first rule is don't become a casualty. So if they tried to kill him, they might try and kill me too. We were stuck there for about an hour and a half, and once or twice we stuck our heads out and were shot at. So I knew."

Bowen and I were in the noisy basement cafeteria of the BBC's offices in White City, London. He was an easy person to talk to, frank in his comments, with a disarming warmth. The interview flowed effortlessly, without the awkward gaps and unspoken tensions that can at times characterize intimate personal revelation. Seven months had passed since the episode he was describing, and the memories were still raw. And like all his colleagues, Bowen clearly displayed the emotional pain involved in retelling traumatic events.

"No one could get to him," he recalled, resuming his story. "So I had to lie low, while my colleague, who was also a good friend, a nice guy, full of jokes, was a hundred yards away, and I didn't know if he was alive or dead. I suspected he was dead. I could see what the shell had done to the car, and I know enough about these things to know that even if flames or shrapnel didn't get you, just being that close to the explosion would give you severe internal injuries that will do you in. And then I knew his family, you see. I had known him, in a sense grown up with him in Lebanon for five years. He was a good guy. He had three children in their teens. I think that for me, the big difference about the tragedy was the personal aspect."

For Bowen the death triggered a cycle of rumination and doubt during which he scrutinized and challenged his actions and judgment. "I was with him, I had just got out of the car myself. If I had stayed, as I easily could have, I would have been killed by the same shell. The thing that affected me as well was that the guy was dead and we stopped there because I said stop there. And then I was not able to help him. At the time it did not seem dangerous to stop there. We thought we were away from the front line, but the tank fired over the border. On the other hand, I know that had I not said let's stop here he might be alive today. But that really is part of the risk that comes with my kind of work. I have sorted it out in my own head, I think. I have replayed it in my mind many times and . . ."

The sentence is left hanging in the air, unfinished, perhaps an indication that no matter how much soul-searching occurs, no matter how detailed the postmortem examination, a sense of guilt can never be fully erased. The tormenting question, What if?—for which no answer can ever prove satisfactory—emerges, challenging the kind of decision that has been made countless times before, over many years of conflict reporting, without adverse consequences, until one day it all goes horribly wrong and one is left in a miasma of self-reproach and remorse. "I have never really had bad dreams," Bowen told me, "but I did after that—successive depressing dreams over a period of about ten days to two weeks. All my friends were dying in the dreams, everyone was dying. So I went to get some counseling." In time, as the sadness, guilt and anger began to wane, Bowen came to realize that there is no real answer to this question. Indeed, the question itself is inherently unfair, as it implies a death that might have been preventable. In the absence of gross negligence or recklessness, such an argument is specious, an insight Bowen was able to articulate.

"I went to Abed's funeral in Beirut, and I was back in south Lebanon the next morning. Someone said to me, 'Have you heard about Kurt [Schork] and Miguel [Moreno]?' I knew both of them very well—they were friends of mine. I said no and was told they had been killed in Sierra Leone the day before. It was the first I had heard of it. And those two days were very nasty. Some friends of mine said we always thought Kurt had this invulnerability about him. I have never thought that, not about Kurt, or about me, not about anybody. There is no magic potion involved in this. Nobody has some *muti* that keeps him protected. If you are there, it is dangerous. And the more you do, the greater the chance of getting it. I mean, how many lives do you have?"

―――――

Why is one journalist killed while another survives? That is one of the great imponderables of this profession. From a psychological perspective, the arbitrariness of fate, luck, chance may also be one of the most powerful determinants of mood, for my data reveal that if loss predicts depression, survival can, in certain circumstances, be the antidote. The reason for this is that when a journalist pulls through after serious injury, his close colleagues are spared an agonizing self-examination that is so often the harbinger of morbid ruminations and low spirits. John Martin's account of an episode during the Yugoslav civil war illustrates this point.

Martin is a veteran television cameraman who has spent more than twenty years in conflict zones. His résumé reads like a who's who of late-twentieth-century warfare. We met for an interview on a rainy summer's day in London, and after running through various symptom checklists, we turned to the topic of one of his more harrowing experiences. "No one had got to the front lines in Vukovar, where the Serbs and Croats were battling," he told me. "I showed up with my soundmen and David Chater, a colleague from ITN, and we managed to use an early morning mist as cover to go down into Vukovar. We went straight through a barrage, the shells and mortars passing across the top of our car, which frightened the life out of the sound guys, who I think had had too much to drink the night before. We managed to get through the roadblocks and into the front lines. Then fortunately or unfortunately we found ourselves tied up with some sort of renegade Serb front-line militia who had been there too long and were already on their first bottle of slivovitz at six o'clock in the morning. They were barking mad Rambo types, with the headbands—you know what I mean. There was heavy incoming fire and we were in a maze of buildings, and around the corner a tank was firing down the street. We were in really deep, to the point that we couldn't get out because the sniping was too accurate. The two front lines were very close, a few yards away from each other, and they were lugging mortars across the street. All the while I had been filming and had some great stuff, also some crazy stuff. Then the Serbs told us they were going to try a breakthrough with some tanks, and did we want to film it? Well, we moved into a church to get close to the tanks, but the attack got bogged down, and we found ourselves under intense fire. It became impossible to get in or out of the church because the Croats were firing rocket-propelled grenades and mortars at the church. I told the team it would be best for us to sit tight for five minutes, during which I would try to repair one of my cameras and then we would head back again. I did my normal thing of getting behind the biggest wall I could and sat down. And then as I was trying to put a lens back on I looked up and just saw David Chater go up in the air and down again. He had stood up, stepped forward in front of a window and a sniper just put one straight through him."

Faced with a seriously wounded colleague, Martin instinctively reached for his camera. "Well, I filmed it—I suppose it's a natural instinct—and then ran across to where he had gone down and the militia put out some covering fire. At this stage there were bodies all over the place, and it was turning into a bloody massacre. We managed to get through the back door, a couple of guys helped us and we dragged him out. I thought David was dead. He had turned that horrible white color and was gushing blood everywhere. The bullet had gone underneath his flak and clean out the other side. Miraculously we managed to find a front-line vehicle that was just ferrying some troops, and we threw him in there, screaming and shouting. The Serbs gave us a ride, and we got him back to a front-line MASH hospital where we did a considerable amount of shouting and finally got him onto a medevac going back and forth to Belgrade. We couldn't go with him. It was a bad scene down there and the medevac was completely full, so we had the two-and-a-half-hour drive to Belgrade, which I didn't enjoy very much—very definitely an unpleasant time because I was pretty much under the theory that when we got to Belgrade I would find a dead reporter friend. But he survived. He was in hospital for three and a half weeks, and the treatment he got was better than you get in the U.K. because they are much better at doing gunshot wounds, as in Belfast."

There are many remarkable aspects to this anecdote: the risks the journalists took in getting to the front lines in Vukovar, the accounts of militiamen drunk at 6 a.m. while waging war, the serious wounding of a colleague, the inability of a flak jacket to keep out the bullet (echoes here of Ken Oosterbroek in the townships of

South Africa, where a bullet again slipped under the jacket, in that case ensuring a fatal outcome), Martin's immediate reaction in filming his stricken colleague, the fortuitous presence of front-line transport, a nearby clearing station and a medevac, the skill of the trauma physicians. From a behavioral standpoint, there is no depression, guilt or heavy drinking, no nightmares, ruminations or flashbacks. The aftermath is fundamentally different from that experienced by Jeremy Bowen and Allan Little because David Chater survived, thereby sparing Martin and his colleagues the agonizing What if? question. Survival—the result of a few millimeters or a couple of seconds. Such are the vagaries confronted by war journalists when they report for work, a confluence of innumerable details often so routine that they hardly penetrate conscious awareness. And it is the interplay of these details, fortunate or adverse, that may also determine the psychological health of the survivors.

Depression is just one of the conditions often found with post-traumatic stress disorder. Substance abuse is another, as Anthony Loyd's memoir makes clear. *My War Gone By: I Miss It So* is an account of the Bosnian war unlike any other. Loyd goes far beyond revealing the brutality of that conflict and the hazards confronted by journalists in getting their story out. He also dwells at length on his addiction to cocaine and alcohol. The title itself reveals Loyd's addictive personality, with the adrenaline rush of war fueling his deep-seated psychological need, akin to a biological craving, for excitement. Away from the front lines, he found the relative dullness of daily life was insufferable and relieved only by the seductive powers of cocaine.

While Loyd's book may illustrate an intemperate case of addictive behavior in a war journalist there are many other examples of colleagues who resort to alcohol or drugs to modulate their environment, either to relieve the mundanity of life in a civil society or to blunt the fear and emotional pain that march in tandem with conflict. One comes away from reading the memoirs of many war journalists with a sense that their world is awash in booze and a pharmacopoeia of illicit and prescription drugs. Tim Page, the famed Vietnam photographer whose behavior and battlefield exploits bear an uncanny resemblance to the character portrayed by Dennis Hopper in Francis Ford Coppola's *Apocalypse Now*, did not spare his reader the details of his substance-abuse problem in his autobiography, *Page After Page: Memoirs of a War-Torn Photographer*. "Everyone was walking around with fluted glass-stopped bottles of Sandoz 25, the purest LSD on the tightening market," he writes. "Traditionally you were given a lump of sugar; I got mine as a splash on my hand, behind the left thumb. I just licked it up. Endlessly." A second anecdote illustrates how a powerful cocktail of barbiturates mixed with alcohol played havoc with his judgment. "Lots of booze, dilaudid, phenobarb and dilantin blurred my pain and desperation. The gun was still with me. The metal glinted purposefully. I got a handful of the hollow-nosed slugs out of the Indian deerskin drawsack and counted out five. The cartridges snick slid home in the chambers, which clicked satisfyingly home in the breech. I spun the barrel and in one movement pointed straight between the eyes and pulled the trigger. My eyes blurred and refocused on the barrel, unsmoking, a black hole, a round in the chamber either side. I lowered the message miracle very slowly and lay back, wiped out." Page's turbulent life is, at times, an extraordinary example of emotions and judgment gone awry, but it is through accounts such as his, Loyd's and many others that drink and drugs have worked their way into the mythology of the war journalist.

The medical complications of alcohol abuse are well known and legion. To assist physicians in monitoring whether their patients are drinking too much, clear guidelines for what constitutes heavy or excessive drinking have been formulated. The upper limit of weekly intake differs for males and females, a reflection of differences in physiology and the ability of the liver to metabolize alcohol. For males the advisable limit is fourteen units a week, for females nine units. A unit is defined as a glass of wine, a shot of spirits or an average-size (11 oz/330 mL) bottle of beer.

My study compared the weekly drinking habits of the 140 war journalists with those from the control group of 107 domestic journalists. Because there are gender differences, the male and female data were analyzed separately. Among the male journalists, those in the war group drank significantly more than the domestic journalists. In fact, the war group's average weekly alcohol consumption was fifteen units, twice that of the domestic journalists, and exceeded the medical guidelines for acceptable drinking. A total of 14 percent of the group drank more than double the weekly limit, while some prodigious individual weekly consumptions were noted—namely, a couple of journalists drinking in excess of two bottles of whisky a week. None of the domestic journalists got close to this level of imbibing.

It is, however, important not to lose sight of the broader perspective, and here some salient observations must be made. First, while male war journalists as a group drink to excess, 59 percent drink fewer than fourteen units a week, and 10 percent of these are virtual teetotalers. It is the remaining 40-plus percent that pushes the average up. Second, the heavy and moderate drinkers showed no greater evidence of depression, post-traumatic stress disorder or overall psychological distress. Thus, excessive alcohol consumption in the war group was not consistent with more extensive psychopathology. Nor was it associated with increased physical problems. A final correlate with respect to males is worth noting: those who drank to excess were significantly more likely to be single or divorced. While the causality of this relationship cannot be stated with certainty, the possibility exists that the most injurious effects of alcohol are in the social domain, with impaired relationships one notable example.

The drinking habits of female war journalists mirror to a degree those of their male counterparts, albeit with the contrasts between the war and domestic groups more pronounced. Their average weekly alcohol consumption of eleven units is well above the cutoff limit of nine units and three times that of the domestic female group. Fifty-two percent of female war journalists were heavy drinkers compared with 41 percent of males and only 7 percent of domestic female journalists. Like their male counterparts, female war journalists whose weekly intake exceeded the cutoff point were not more likely to endorse symptoms of depression, PTSD, psychological distress or physical illness. However, the genders diverged when it came to marital status; female heavy drinkers were just as likely to be married as those who tended toward moderation.

The reactions of those in the profession to these findings were interesting. War journalists and their news bosses listened respectfully to the PTSD and depression data, but the information on alcohol and its interpretation within rigid medical orthodoxy prompted howls of laughter and occasionally outright derision. Many war journalists are hard drinking; they know it and in a macho way are proud of it. They certainly have little patience for a behavioral scientist with his cutoff thresholds, pedantic definitions and measuring cup. I had a sense that they greeted my empirical data with much the same enthusiasm as that shown by a publican for a Salvation Army prohibitionist.

Within war zones, shortages of food and water may exist alongside a thriving black market well supplied with liquor. And here alcohol fulfills many roles. Recall John Martin's account of Serb and Croat militia tanked up on slivovitz at 6 a.m. and fighting with reckless abandon. Or the words of a bereaved journalist, mourning the death of a close colleague: "I drank a lot . . . and drugs had always been part of the scene anyway. . . . I was very self-destructive." Or journalists hunkered down at night in a war zone, unable to venture outdoors, with nothing but a bottle to help pass the time and assist as a hypnotic. There have, of course, been circumstances in which liquor was hard to come by. Afghanistan, for example, presented the fraternity with challenges that, to some,

seemed more daunting than personal danger. The unyielding impo-
sition of Islamic fundamentalism had effectively turned the country into a dry state. A month into the post–September 11 American
bombing campaign, the *Times* of London ran an article by the
dauntless and entertaining Anthony Loyd entitled "Death and
Moonshine." Loyd speaks for many when he describes war as a
combination of the "thrilling rush of excitement followed by the
backwash of boredom," and while there is little he can do to influence the former, addressing the latter falls well within his repertoire. "Alcohol is a very underground scene," he wrote. "There
are a few networks still in place, principally among isolated phar-
macists. They need alcohol to make medicine and a few diversify.
[The homemade liquor they sell] tastes like grappa. If you mix the
clear liquid with fruit juice imported over the passes on mule trains
from Pakistan and Iran, the result isn't bad, though the joy of our
first test run was spoilt by fears of imminent blindness. To work
out the quality you pour a drop on wood and try to light it. If it
lights with a blue flame you are in luck: if not, then the grog's been
cut with meat fat and you've been ripped off."

A humorous interlude, but one that is nevertheless revealing.
For Loyd and Seamus, his freelancer photographer friend, the illicit
brew offered a way of passing the slow, dark Afghan nights. Others
may use alcohol for different reasons. For some war journalists, the
sights, smells and sounds of war are never entirely banished; they
return unexpectedly, at awkward moments, like some unwelcome
guest crashing a party. Initially, alcohol may offer respite, an effective, albeit short-lived anodyne, the powerful suppressant effects of
a stiff drink blotting out the intrusive, nightmarish demons of involuntary recollection. But tolerance can set in, and soon what one
drink once achieved now requires two, or three or four. Alcohol also
makes a bad sleeping draft, because it disrupts the rhythms of sleep.
In time, an easy solution becomes very much part of the problem.

Donatella Lorch is currently a national correspondent for *Newsweek*. While a reporter for the *New York Times*, she covered wars in

Somalia, Sudan, Afghanistan, Rwanda and Zaire, among others. In an article entitled "Surviving the Five Ds," she recalled how her work centered on covering the Dead, the Dying, the Diseased, the Depressing and the Dangerous. It is a heartfelt article, describing the elation and sorrow of life as a war journalist, and it touches on many of the themes addressed thus far, including the alienation felt on returning home ("For those few months back in the United States, I struggled with an emptiness that I nursed alone at night in my darkened living room, watching the lights of New Jersey across the Hudson River, wine in hand, deeply lonely, anxious and unhappy"); the habituation to the horrors of war ("We joked about dead bodies over sushi at a Japanese restaurant in Nairobi, much to the shock of the neighboring tables"), the unconscious re-experiencing of trauma-related memories ("If smell can trigger memories, all I need is to catch a whiff of road kill before I remember the churches of Rwanda and the hills of Burundi"), her hypervigilance and that of colleagues ("Even living in Rome, he felt apprehension—scanning the roads around him, looking for snipers, avoiding untraveled routes. Even now I catch myself, for brief moments, looking for danger, wary of walking on unmarked trails because of landmines or just checking people out to see if anyone looks suspicious").

Insightful as her article is, I would respectfully add one more D to her somber list: drink. It runs like a thread through her brief narrative, from watching the lights of the Hudson alone in her apartment, glass of wine in hand, to her observations of colleagues ("I have watched many drink heavily and at least one slip into alcoholism") and her memories of Mogadishu ("We drank heavily, many smoked dope, at least one did hard drugs"). She also takes issue with the findings of my study, writing that "[a]ccording to a Freedom Forum–sponsored study, female war journalists drink five times as much as their counterparts in the general journalistic population. I do drink more than before I went to Africa, but I would like to think that it would probably compare to a European

male counterpart's consumption." There is an element of defi-
ance, if not pride, in her assertion that as a female she has an ability
to knock them back that is the equal of any male colleague's. And
to reinforce her point, she refers specifically to the European male,
with the tacit understanding that liberal drinking habits in the Old
World are very much part of the social fabric of everyday life,
unlike in North America, where such behavior elicits a pejorative
response. To which I can reply that she is correct on all points,
save one. Female war journalists can drink as heavily as their male
colleagues, but this should be cause for consternation, not pride.
When concern is expressed over alcohol consumption (for both
genders) it should not be viewed as some preachy reprimand
implying personal failure. There is no simply no question that
drinking to excess is bad for your health.

For an empiricist, the findings seem clear enough. But I'll add
one final caveat that illustrates the difficulties of drawing simple
conclusions. For the majority of war journalists, alcohol has not
impeded their ability to write, film, televise and produce with skill
and creativity, often under uncommonly difficult circumstances. If
it is important to recognize the medical risks of heavy long-term
drinking, it is also important to acknowledge that for many war
journalists the symbiosis of drink and work fits poorly with a conventional wisdom captured by Oscar Wilde's witticism that work
is the curse of the drinking class.

———

Data were also collected with respect to other forms of substance
abuse—namely, the use of cannabis, cocaine, barbiturates, LSD
and opiates. The cannabis findings were analyzed separately
because the assumption was that it would be fairly common in
both groups of journalists, as it is in the general population, and
therefore less likely to represent socially maladaptive behavior.
This hypothesis was proved correct. Twenty-four percent of war

journalists and 19 percent of domestic journalists used cannabis on a regular basis, a difference that was not statistically significant. When it came to other drugs, 6 percent of war journalists and 2 percent of domestic journalists reported using them, cocaine being the most frequently cited drug. These relatively small percentages reveal that hard-drug abuse is not common. Chasing the dragon is confined to a small minority, with the profession as a whole wary of highly addictive and dangerous substances.

Given that alcohol and drug abuse often go together, I looked at hard-drug use among those deemed to be either "average" or "excessive" drinkers. This analysis was confined to males, as only two female journalists were hard-drug users. The results showed that those males who drank to excess were also the ones using cocaine and, to a lesser extent, amphetamines and LSD.

There is a class of medication, the benzodiazepines (Valium is an example) that make good sleeping pills. Most journalists are well aware of their sedating, calming effects, but they are less familiar with the problems associated with prolonged use. As with alcohol, the potential for addiction is high and self-medicating is ill advised. However, when a journalist is far from the safety of home and circumstances fray the nerves, the temptation to dip into the bottle is hard to resist. Fergal Keane described the enticing pull of an anesthetic sleep amid the stench of death in Rwanda. "I'd brought some sleeping pills with me because people who had advice on Rwanda were telling me it was crazy," he told me. "We were stuck in this place. We had almost driven into an ambush that day. We were driving down a road and saw two men with AK47s on their backs placing a mine on the road. We managed to turn around and drive back. We then had to take a short-cut through country that was crawling with these characters. We had seen what they had done and it was the thought of falling victim to them. . . . We eventually arrived that night in a village that was just full of dead bodies. There was a small detachment of the guerrilla army, the good guys, in the village, and we went over to say hello. They were edgy and knew they could be attacked at any moment. That night we sat around in a tiny hut, passing around pictures of our families. And I said, I've got some sleeping pills, because there was no way we were going to sleep. The smell of the corpses was just overpowering. So we took sleeping pills that night and they wiped us out."

The situation is exacerbated by the fact that Valium has a street value—vast quantities often flood zones of conflict, making its procurement easy and cheap. One cameraman recalled that during his time in Sarajevo, "I was taking a lot of sedatives. I had a bag of two thousand Valium. Somebody was just handing them out. They had been given to him by the French [peacekeepers] because he had been in a TV station that had been hit by a shell. So I remember eating a lot of Valium, getting stoned, drinking. Somehow through that I was working as well because there wasn't any down time, only a couple of hours' sleep here and there. Everything was just spiraling out of control."

———

This chapter has laid out the prevalence of alcohol abuse and the use of hard drugs among war journalists. It is the first attempt at providing empirical evidence to complement or counterbalance the many anecdotes that fill this profession's genre of turbulent autobiography. To what extent do these two realities match up? Are the objective findings in concordance with the personal revelations? The answer, not surprisingly, depends on who is viewing the data.

From the perspective of the behavioral scientist, the addition of a control group, in this instance domestic journalists carefully screened to ensure they had never so much as sniffed the winds of war, was an essential prerequisite. This provided the means to statistically interpret the data and assign clinical relevance. With this design in place, the results are unequivocal. War journalists drink more heavily and show an inclination toward more illicit drug use, particularly cocaine. These are telling observations, yet when they're reduced to the objectivity of medical diagnoses, they take on a disembodied quality. What this dry taxonomy translates into is this: the lives of some war journalists are, at times, clouded by nightmares, flashbacks, eidetic images of death and destruction, emotional detachment, fraught relationships, sadness, guilt, thoughts of suicide and periods of intense loneliness. Getting drunk and perhaps getting stoned offer temporary relief. Rather than bringing succor, though, this behavior, if sustained, introduces a fresh set of problems while aggravating old difficulties.

But we must remember that if 29 percent of war journalists develop PTSD over the course of a lifetime, that leaves 70-plus percent who do not, which goes with the 76 percent who do not develop major depression, the 60 percent who do not drink heavily and the 94 percent who decline the laced fluted glass. Depression-free war journalists who drink moderately and avoid drugs are quick to point out that generalizations are frequently misleading. They can cite angst-free memoirs, like those of John Simpson and Sandy Gall, that reveal a more moderate side to the profession. This argument too has a legitimacy.

Perhaps the most accurate and fairest summation of the many variables in my data set is this: the extent to which war journalists use alcohol, barbiturates and cocaine lies along a continuum, with the exploits of Tim Page and Anthony Loyd at one end and the 10 percent of teetotaling, acid-free journalists at the other. Between them come the bulk of their colleagues whose predilections nevertheless exceed those of their domestic counterparts and the general population. The war journalist data are thus out of kilter, shifted off center, away from the norms of society at large. Given the nature of their work, this is perhaps not surprising. These findings must be cause for concern, but it would be a mistake to pathologize so large a majority, for I have no evidence showing that their work suffers as a consequence of this behavior and only the weakest, inferential data suggesting relationships are adversely impacted. It is these observations, empirically supported, rather than the incandescent prose of a tempestuous memoir, that more accurately reflect the profession's complex flirtation with addiction.

5

FREELANCE WAR JOURNALISTS: GOING SOLO INTO ZONES OF CONFLICT

The strongest man in the world is he who stands most alone

— HENRIK IBSEN

On September 27, 2002, the London *Times* ran an obituary titled "British TV Man Killed in Chechen Battle." The article, which angered the small community of freelance journalists, reported that "the British author of a travel guide to the world's most dangerous places has been killed as Chechen rebels fought a fierce battle against an overwhelming Russian force." The man in question, Gervaise Roderick "Roddy" John Scott, was found dead alongside eighty Chechen fighters killed by Russian artillery and air attacks. Russian television reported that he died when a bullet pierced the lens of his camera: a picture of the shattered lens and smashed Nikon supported the claim. Roddy Scott was thirty-one years of age.

What particularly angered Vaughan Smith, the director of a freelance agency, Frontline Television News, were certain of the assertions made in the *Times* obituary. Rather than concentrating on the quality of Scott's journalism, the authors saw fit to play up his contributions to an annual travel guide, *The World's Most Dangerous Places*, mentioning that he had once spent time "cooling his heels in an Ethiopian jail," and that he chose to "seek out the least visited or most dangerous spots, and then manage[d] to choose the world's most dangerous people to travel with." Moving between innuendo and frank claims of reckless and potentially self-injurious behavior, the obituarists quoted a nameless colleague who labeled Scott's desire to cover the war in Chechnya as "practically suicidal and really crazy. There's this bandit, outlaw connection. You could be kidnapped. The Russians might shoot you. The rebels might shoot you. There's no safe side for you if you are a Western journalist in Chechnya."

Reading the faint and damning praise in the *Times*, one comes away with little sense of Roddy Scott's worth. What is left is an uncomfortable feeling that a combination of extreme sensation-seeking behavior and a cavalier and foolish bravado has, inevitably, brought about his tragic end.

However, a subsequent obituary, published in the Toronto *Globe and Mail* and written by another colleague of Scott's, paints a very different picture. The man who looks out from the pages of the *Globe*, his youthful, open gaze inserted beside a blurry enlarged photograph of his destroyed camera, is remembered as a charismatic figure, intrepid, inquiring, devoted to telling the story of the world's forgotten conflicts. Forsaking financial reward, undaunted by the risk of nasty infectious diseases (while reporting the civil war in Sierra Leone, Scott had contracted cerebral malaria and temporarily lost his sight), he had ventured repeatedly into territory, both geographical and abstract, that many other war journalists avoided, befriending the local people and their militias, gaining their trust and respect and in the process telling a compelling and articulate story that the world's news organizations were increasingly reluctant to hear. The tone of the article differs markedly from that expressed in the *Times*, for the Canadian obituary, filled with affection and admiration, eulogizes Scott, celebrating a remarkable life while mourning the premature demise of a journalist whose work combined the rare attributes of courage and selflessness.

Two such radically different perspectives on a life short lived. In tallying the qualities and content of a man's life such a posthumous falling out is more the legacy of veteran politicians than a little-known thirty-one-year-old cameraman, killed along the border of Chechnya and Ingushetia. That the individual in question was a freelance journalist, however, hints at a fault line that runs through the profession, a divide separating the self-employed from those working on contract to the news networks. "What is clear is that many in the media still feel uncomfortable with real freelancers," wrote Vaughan Smith, three days after his colleague's death. "Of course, the *Times* would write differently of one of their own or any journalist working for any mainstream media organization. Did they write this when the foreign correspondent for the *Sunday Times*, Marie Colvin, lost an eye in Sri Lanka?"

What lay behind Smith's ardent defense of his colleague and freelancers in general was more than a grievance over cynical double standards. It reflected his passionate belief in the importance of reportage cut loose from the control of news organizations with their myriad competing agendas. A credo of the freelance journalist, one of the common denominators that bind this group and give their work an added significance, is independence of spirit, tethered as it can be to moral rectitude. "Roddy felt the international media was in dereliction of its duty in failing to take the necessary risks to cover Chechnya," wrote Smith. He believed that freelancers were the only ones willing to report on conflicts that the mainstream media, out of fear or political bias, wanted to ignore.

Independence does, however, have its own weighty demands. James Nachtwey articulates a philosophy shared by the thirty freelancers who were part of my study. "If you really want to establish yourself and show that you mean business and you're serious about it, you sometimes have to do an assignment on your own.

You may have just enough money in the bank to make it through the trip, speculating on whether you'll ever recover your expenses and break even.... I've done that a number of times.... I continue to do that, and I think it's a mark of the fact that I'm very serious about what I'm doing, that it means something to me and I don't just wait for an assignment."

Certainly, the career path described by Nachtwey isn't the road to riches. In praising the virtues of Roddy Scott, Vaughan Smith lays out, in stark detail, the meager earnings his friend could count on. "The remarkable thing about Roddy was that he was able to get into Chechnya, having waited in Georgia for several months, on a budget of just £500. His trip was delayed for three months while he waited for a broadcaster to pay us for two minutes of Afghan footage sold for £250 per minute earlier this year. We laughed with him as we handed over the £500 before he set off, when he told us he hoped he would get film so compelling that he'd be paid enough to buy a new pair of boots."

Vaughan Smith's criticism is directed primarily at the management of the major news organizations, but he is not the only one to have spelled out the tensions between the different categories of journalists. Mark Pedelty is an anthropologist who went to El Salvador during that country's civil war to study the Salvadoran Foreign Press Corps Association (SPECA). A chapter in his book *War Stories: The Culture of Foreign Correspondents* offers a detailed comparison of staff journalists employed by the news networks and stringers (self-employed local journalists who sell articles, radio pieces and photos to a number of news organizations, called "strings").* He writes that stringers harbor a great deal of animosity toward staff correspondents, whom they call the A Team. The

---

* While the term "stringers" is generally reserved for persons hired *on* location in zones of conflict, as opposed to freelancers who are hired to go *to* a location, there may be considerable overlap in what these journalists do and in the terms of their employment.

litany of complaints from the B Team includes the following: the A Team is physically and culturally removed from the conflict; the A Team exploits the B Team's knowledge without adequate compensation; the A Team is too closely linked to elite, propagandistic sources of information (a. k. a. the American State Department) and receives preferential treatment in return. Pedelty, whose sympathies in El Salvador clearly lay with the stringers, contrasts the objective reporting and intellectual independence of the freelancers with the A Team's excessive obedience to their organization, their piety akin to political toadyism.

According to Pedelty, stringers refer to the latter as the *New York Times* disease, a nefarious condition whose symptoms include journalists defining themselves by the organization they work for, while the organization in turn defines what constitutes the news ("If the *Times* isn't there, it isn't news"). Reading Pedelty's monograph is like discovering a war within a war. The *New York Times* disease is described as "a virulent hubris more common than its label implies," and while the author acknowledges that some of the stringers' accusations are extreme and driven in part by envy, he also paints an unattractive portrait of the staff correspondents. These exponents of "parachute journalism" appear crassly manipulative, short on empathy, driven by narcissism, almost psychopathic in their exploitation and manipulation of people. And to cap it all, they "participate conspicuously in prostitution." In one of those awful psychologist-manqué attempts at insight, Pedelty explains this unsavory sexual predilection thus: "Following the tradition of war correspondents past, they construct their professional identities through sexual adventure. Furthermore, through such adventures they recoup a sense of power, compensating for that which is ceded daily to censoring (neutering?) structures. In other words, they may not be allowed to write like Mr. Hemingway, but they can at least attempt to live like him. Therefore, it is only natural that the world's oldest profession would intersect with one of its most frustrating."

It is unfortunate that the foreign correspondent who emerges from Pedelty's pages is at times closer to caricature, for his study is the first and most detailed social examination of the profession. Nevertheless, embedded within his distorted profile are certain truths that define the differences between foreign journalists and their freelance counterparts, and it is these that resonate with Vaughan Smith's more composed assessment. "I wouldn't want to give the impression that real freelancers don't have friends in the industry," he writes. "We have very many and are very grateful to them. You only have to look at the list of those who support the Rory Peck Trust—a charity to support the wider television freelance community, set up in the name of a real freelancer killed in 1993 —each year to see that we are appreciated. Indeed Roddy completed a safety course that was part funded by the trust. But few of those in our industry who wish us well have ever quite understood us. Think awhile what was going through Roddy's mind as he set off with Chechen rebels. As a single man, he didn't worry about insurance, though he would have welcomed it. Nor did he miss the flak jacket he couldn't afford on his £500 budget."

Unlike agency journalists, freelancers lack support and backup should they get into difficulties, which they often can't avoid, given the nature of their work and the places visited. The benefits of working for a news agency, such as life insurance, armored vehicles for transport in and out of areas of conflict and help on the other end of a telephone line, are eschewed in favor of independence, the choice of deciding what to do, where to go and what to record, unfettered by the constraints of the news bosses and an imposed political agenda. Gary Knight, a freelance photographer married to a network journalist, deftly summarized their different work conditions. "During the war in Bosnia, my wife, Fiona, and I would often make our separate ways to the field. Fiona, a TV producer, would leave the house in a silver limousine, with $10,000 to $20,000 in her bag, armed with pages of research. She would fly in business class and be greeted upon arrival by a local producer, who would have arranged her onward travel and would brief her fully on the current situation. Fiona would work for two or three weeks in the field, traveling in an armored car with her crew and correspondent, communicating by satellite telephone, with practically everything she needed at her disposal. When she returned home, in the same elegant manner as she left, she could even get counseling and medical care, if needed.

"I, on the other hand, was totally on my own. During the war in Yugoslavia, some magazines would give freelancers only guarantees, not assignments. That way they could not be held responsible if a photographer was killed or wounded. Guarantees never covered expenses, however. So, shortly after Fiona left, I would head for the airport in the cheapest taxi available, raiding an ATM brave enough to accept my card. I would take a cheap flight and, on arrival, would hire a cheap, 'soft-skinned' car and make my way to the story. If things got hot along the way, I would put the car seat in maximum recline and drive as fast as I could. If I needed to speak to the magazine client, I would first have to find a satellite phone. In Sarajevo, that meant driving down Sniper Alley in full recline. Once I got in phone contact with the magazine, I would be kept on hold for ten minutes. That cost $450. My overnight accommodation was usually on someone else's floor. By the end of some of these trips, I would arrive home having spent more money than I had earned."

The differences between these two groups belie the fact that they often need each other. The freelancers' much-cherished independence ends when it comes to getting their work before the public, while the news organizations may look to them to provide content. So begins an uneasy, enforced symbiosis amid often divergent agendas. These tensions are magnified when a freelance journalist is wounded or killed. Many of the journalists I interviewed gave examples of how a news organization that had been keen to purchase their material suddenly dropped from sight when they were in trouble. When the plane in which John Liebenberg was traveling was shot down over Huambo in central Angola, he suddenly confronted just such a reality. "It was then that I got really pissed at Reuters," he told me. "Reuters never contacted my family. Reuters knew we had gone down. There was a plane flying above us, and those guys in the plane saw the aircraft going down and immediately put it on the wires. We, the survivors, were stuck on the front lines for fourteen days. When I got out of that hole, I took it up with them, but they just kept quiet. They never answered anything. I was really angry with them. Reuters has that ability to do that to people. They will warn you, John, watch out for the dangers and the consequences, but we want the pictures. And when you are putting your ass on the line, and you get knocked out, hurt, they'll ask you, John, didn't you take too many chances? Are you sure it was the right decision you took? It made me a little shaky. Because I wanted to come back to my work, I wanted to come back to my children, I wanted to be alive and I wanted to be a father."

The photographer Greg Marinovich tells of a similar experience in his memoir *The Bang-Bang Club*. "The reason for my unease about working with *Newsweek* as opposed to *Time* was one of corporate culture. I felt unsure that *Newsweek* were the right people to back me up in what was a potentially dangerous story: in Bosnia I had done work on guarantee for *Newsweek*, covering the Muslim-Croat conflict, a nasty war where a drive along a valley road saw you cross front lines several times and I came to experience the difference between *Newsweek*'s attitude and that of their great rival, *Time*. I had asked if I could hire a 'hard car'—bulletproofed vehicle that would dramatically increase my safety, and give me an advantage in getting pictures. *Newsweek*'s answer was no; they suggested I get a ride with someone who had a hard car. This meant asking Nachtwey, the *Time* photographer, if I could ride with him. When *Time* assigns a photographer to a war zone they make sure there is as little extra pressure put on them as possible. They spend money to get the best pictures and safeguard their photographers, even if they are just freelancers.

"An assignment is an agreement to temporarily employ you on a fixed day rate, pay all your expenses and accept responsibility for you in case something happens. *Newsweek*'s method was to give freelance photographers a guarantee that would cover expenses, day rates and car hire. The guarantee system could put a few dollars more in your pocket if you stayed in cheap hotels and skimped on expenses. It was quite different to being on assignment. The system of guarantees had evolved as a hands-off way of getting photographs. The company is allegedly less liable if someone gets hurt or killed while on guarantee than if that person is on assignment. Photograph-lore has it that *Newsweek* had instituted that system after photographers working for them had been expensively hurt or killed."

Soon Marinovich had an opportunity to see for himself if the rumors about *Newsweek* were true. While covering the township violence that preceded the 1994 elections in South Africa, he was seriously wounded. "I would discover that my unease about working for that magazine was well founded," he wrote. "They did not offer one day's pay for the weeks in hospital or the months of recuperation." When we met, six years had passed since Marinovich's shooting, and his views of the news organizations remained uncompromising. "Most of them are just exploitative," he asserted. "*Time* magazine is one of the few that isn't. . . . The last day *Newsweek* paid me was the day I was shot. I was on assignment for them. I was on contract. They paid my little bills. They paid no compensation. Nothing else. And they kept promising, instead of which they never delivered. And I was in such a fucked-up state that I just went along with everything. I kept on asking for help and they just kept evading. Listen, it's a business. It's taken me a long time to discover that, but it's a business. Nothing more, nothing less."

Being judged exploitative and callously indifferent does not sit well with the news bosses. I asked Stephen Jukes, the global head of news at Reuters, to clarify what had happened to Liebenberg in Angola, but he drew a blank—the episode in question had taken place too far in the past for anyone currently working at Reuters to remember the details. Jukes did, however, provide me with a list of safety procedures and policies that his organization had implemented for freelance journalists. These include providing insurance in the event of death or long-term disability. Freelancers are also sent on hostile-environment training. Furthermore, Jukes made it clear that Reuters is aware that the intense competitive pressures among freelance cameramen in war zones may inadvertently push them to take greater risks. To mitigate this, Reuters and other large news networks have agreed to pool material in situations of extreme danger. Jukes also cited specific cases of the highest rungs of management in his organization intervening when tragedy and danger overtook one of their freelancers. When Kurt Schork was killed in Sierra Leone in 2000, for example, Reuters worked with his family in making the funeral arrangements, which involved repatriating his body from West Africa. Reuters also helped establish the Kurt Schork Memorial Fund.

The story with respect to the allegations against *Newsweek* was in many respects similar. The photographer Gary Knight related how the current management was more safety conscious and had recently sent him on a nuclear, biological and chemical warfare training course. He did, however, acknowledge that back in the early 1990s, when Marinovich and the Bang-Bang Club were combing the dusty, lethal alleys of the South African townships for photographs, management was more indifferent to their fate.

In a profession where death, injury and illness are unavoidable, the business Marinovich refers to is a complicated one. News networks must ask themselves if, by purchasing material from freelance journalists, they are endorsing a work ethic that on occasion places the journalist in grave danger. Is there not a moral responsibility tacit in this financial transaction? If freelance journalists are the only ones prepared to risk their lives to get a particular story, and the news organizations want that story, can these organizations turn their backs on the journalists when they are injured or worse? "We present an ethical problem that comes to the fore when one of us is killed," wrote Vaughan Smith in his obituary for Roddy Scott. Of course, the news organizations could dispense with any moral ambiguity and banish guilt by refusing to buy material from freelance journalists, citing unacceptable risk-taking behavior. But that opens up another issue: should it be the prerogative of the news organizations to define which stories can and cannot be told, which war is important and which one can be ignored?

Dramatic war footage will always prove irresistible to news organizations. Not only are the images riveting, but they often have the additional allure of political, and even historical, importance. Take Roddy Scott's last video, for example. Found on the battlefield by Russian forces, it shows Chechen rebels crossing from Pankisi to north Ossetia and then into Ingushetia, providing incontrovertible evidence that Georgian territory was being used as a springboard for their attacks on Russian forces. According to the *Guardian* newspaper, the footage was shown on Russian television and outraged officials in Moscow.

The discomfort of the news organizations, enticed by the image, yet nervous of the obligations that come with ownership, is unlikely to be assuaged by Vaughan Smith's claim that freelancers "have never asked for anything more than a market to sell to." By absolving news organizations of any responsibility for the physical well-being of freelancers, he deftly usurps the moral high ground. Failing to assist a wounded journalist or washing their hands of the corpse while simultaneously using that journalist's material is callous. To publicly justify doing so by quoting Smith's plaintive plea adds a caddish element to behavior that is already questionable. Smith's high-flown sentiment might clarify where freelance cameramen stand in their business dealings, but it can only have added to the moral burden of those who buy their product. This may be one of the reasons why freelancers are having greater difficulty selling their work. Smith recalls "the good old days when television newsrooms were inhabited by stalwarts such as the BBC's John Mahoney, who not only clearly liked dealing with colorful mavericks like Rory Peck, but also gave us a fair price for our footage. We got £700 per minute. Ten years ago, if you were good, you could match the wage of a BBC reporter. Now we are lucky to get £300 per minute, and there is much more reluctance to purchase in the first place. Broadcasters are now troubled by us."

Another problem is that the interests of a freelance journalist, such as a forgotten war in Angola or conflict in the recesses of the Caucasus, may not mesh with the priorities of a large news organization. This tale of frustration was one I heard repeatedly in my interviews with the freelancers. "I had a really difficult trip to the Congo," the freelance cameraperson Elizabeth Jones told me. "I spent all my own money just to get these images, and I could not find a spot for them." Her terse summary of her months in central Africa was echoed by similar comments from journalists who had worked in Sierra Leone, the Sudan, Mozambique, the Ivory Coast, Somalia, Chechnya, Colombia—a Third World montage of civil collapse and cheap death. With the attention of the developed nations and their well-resourced press corps focused firmly on Afghanistan, the Middle East and the Balkans, it has been left to the "mavericks" to cover the world's unnoticed wars, often at their own expense.

———

Navigating solo war's fickle, lethal uncertainties adds a new dimension of stress and uncertainty and raises the question how this group of journalists fares psychologically. Of the 140 war journalists I studied, 30 were freelance and their responses on the various questionnaires were compared with those given by their network colleagues. My first observation was that freelance journalists are generally younger than their tenured colleagues, although there are some notable exceptions. This fits with theories we've already discussed, linking younger age with more adventurous and physically demanding actions. Freelancers were not, however, more likely to develop PTSD or show more prominent symptoms of the disorder. Thus, while they travel to more inhospitable and dangerous places, this exposure does not translate into more nightmares, flashbacks, startle responses and the like. One reason may be that the degree of violence confronted by all war journalists, freelance or not, is so extreme that teasing out various gradations of PTSD response is not possible. Another possibility is that freelancers, a self-selected group, have an innate ability to better withstand the negative effects of overwhelming violence. This is not to say they are immune to syndromes like PTSD, but relatively speaking their greater exposure to life-threatening events does not translate into more severe or frequent symptoms.

There are two areas where freelance journalists were found to function more poorly. On the General Health Questionnaire, which is a composite measure of psychological distress, they endorsed significantly more symptoms of depression and social dysfunction. The simplest explanation for this is that financial worries, anxieties over selling work, inadequate or absent life insurance, sleeping on floors, bumming lifts, scrounging satellite phones—in short, all the impediments of a stand-alone existence—exert their own toll. Freelance journalists choose this route from conviction. Principles can prove costly, however, as these data show.

Even in death, their position as loners, operating outside established and conventional channels, can be exploited. An ignominious sequel to Roddy Scott's ending makes the point. While colleagues in London sought to counteract the tenet of the *Times* obituary, away in the Caucasus there surfaced controversy of a more ominous nature, this one also fuelled by a journalist's steadfast determination to pursue a story he considered important. The director of the secret service in Ingushetia refused permission for Scott to be buried in the region. The authorities considered him a terrorist. The British embassy was not planning to send a representative, citing security fears. Five weeks after his death, Scott's body still lay in a morgue outside the city of Nazran, denied the dignity of a decent burial. The violent manner in which he had lost his life had not given way to quiet grief or calm reflection.

Courageous reporting may win plaudits, but it also makes for powerful enemies. It is here that the vulnerability of the freelance journalist is once again laid bare. Stripped by injury or death of a formidable self-reliance, he has little protection against slander, imputation and the humiliation of having malevolent apparatchiks deny him a final resting place.

———

Thus far I have confined my comments to freelance journalists who travel to zones of conflict on foreign soil. One thing they have in common with journalists employed by the large news networks is the opportunity to leave war behind and return home for rest, if needed. From my conversations with freelancers, it emerged that the average length of time spent in a war zone was approximately two to three months. At that point, the journalist's body and mind begin emitting unmistakable signs that a rest away from the front lines is needed. Fatigue, insomnia, irritability, edginess take over, or it may be a vague foreboding of doom, often nothing more tangible than a sense of having tempted fate once too often. Jon Jones described this moment as follows: "I remember waking up in the morning—I had been in Sarajevo for fourteen weeks—and thinking, I've got to go. And within ten minutes I set off in a car. I drove from Sarajevo to Vienna without a break. I got on a plane in Vienna and went home. There was this very strong intuitive feeling that I had to go. The trick is to be able to do it and not regret anything you missed during the day. You need to recognize this feeling and not be bothered by the macho kind of bullshit that says, 'Well, I stayed longer than you' and all that crap. The seriously good people will just say, 'I'm going home,' and not care what anyone thinks." Sometimes it was a particular event that made Jones or one of his colleagues reach for the return ticket. "We were driving through the streets of Sarajevo. We stopped, and a tank fired at us and blew the door off the car I was in. It was slightly open. Blew it right off its hinges. So I thought, Oh God, there's a message in this. It was time to leave. Because your time is up. You go with a big bucket of luck and the longer you stay, the more it drips out."

I never did interview a war journalist who did not take a break at some point and return home for a brief period. As disconnected as many journalists often feel back in London or Madrid, a reprieve from snipers, ambushes and ubiquitous death can settle frazzled nerves and calm the spirit. No such respite is possible for those journalists who live in the zones of conflict. Occasionally, they will be hired as stringers by Western news organizations. More often than not the protracted brutality of what is most frequently a civil war rapidly outdistances the limited attention span of the news networks and their viewers. Yet, for the journalists living in these regions, the war is not forgotten. How can it be when the conflict defines daily existence? So the task falls to them and a tiny group of freelance journalists like Roddy Scott to bring news of war to those living through it, and perhaps, with the foresight of an enlightened editor, to those in more distant affluent lands as well.

From a research perspective, a second question now presents itself. How do journalists trapped by war within their own society, and with no chance of respite, fare psychologically? Are the depression and social dysfunction exhibited by freelance journalists magnified by circumstances that hold local journalists captive? Unfortunately, this was not a question my data could answer because there were no local stringers in my sample of 140 war journalists. But I was able to witness, in a less formal way, some of the many adversities confronted by two local journalists working independently in the Third World.

In presenting my account of what I observed, I have no empirical data from which to draw conclusions. My interactions with these two journalists were fundamentally different from those I had with the freelancers and involved intense, daily contact instead of questionnaires and brief interviews. We would meet for breakfast, lunch, dinner. I met one journalist's wife and got to talk with their children and siblings. I visited their offices and spoke with colleagues. Rating scales, with their inbuilt cultural and linguistic biases, would not have been appropriate in this setting. Anecdote and personal observation, therefore, inform my opinion.

In 2001 I took part in a panel discussion in Washington, D.C., with John Owen of the Freedom Forum, Chris Cramer and Mike Hanna of CNN and Donatella Lorch of *Newsweek*. The topic was journalists and safety. When we came to the question-and-answer segment, a middle-aged African man rose from his seat in the darkened auditorium and introduced himself: "Bart Kakooza, Media Plus, Uganda." He blinked into the lights, paused to collect himself and cleared his throat. "Why is it, Doctor," he began, directing his question to me, "that I cannot eat meat? It has been that way ever since I returned from Rwanda. I don't have a problem with other food, but when it comes to meat . . ." His question trailed off. He shrugged and gave an awkward laugh. "I have this problem with meat."

It was one of those moments during public speaking that I have always disliked. Self-revelatory questions such as these are difficult because they divulge only part of the information required to formulate a sensible answer. The questioner, meanwhile, stands expectantly in front of hundreds of people whose attention has suddenly been seized by the dramatic disclosure. They too expect an answer. If that is not challenge enough, you have at most only a couple of minutes in which to reply coherently.

My solution, when faced with such odds, has always been to acknowledge the distress implicit in the question, provide a brief, generic statement alluding to the complex nature of such phenomena and invite the questioner to come up to me after the symposium and discuss the matter further, and in private. Which is what I did in this case. Three weeks later, I found myself on a plane to

Kampala. Bart Kakooza's question, the one that had so riveted the audience's attention, had moved Tom Johnson, chairman and CEO of CNN, to underwrite the cost of sending me to Uganda to come up with a treatment plan.

———————

There was confusion on the ground at the Entebbe terminal. It was late evening and staff were tired. Some travelers had visas, others did not and were shunted off to one side. A few tourists suddenly became aware that a vaccination against yellow fever was required. They stood anxiously in the lineup for passport control, whispering, wondering if they would be allowed into the country. I produced my vaccination record. The customs officer ignored it and waved me through. Bart Kakooza was not waiting for me. He had been called away to cover a story in the Sudan and had instead sent his brother, Deus Akambikira, and a colleague with the unlikely name of Henry Ford.

Henry was hobbling on crutches. We made our way to their parked car, and I settled in for the ride into Kampala. It was dark and I could make out little of the surrounding countryside, for there are no street lights. We exchanged pleasantries about my flight, and I asked Henry about his leg. I had not noticed a cast so had assumed the injury was slight—a twisted ankle, perhaps, or a bruised knee. But I was wrong, and Henry began his tale of woe, a story unlike any other I had heard. It was a story that would unfold over the course of the week I spent in the verdant hills of Kampala and involved not only Henry but his wife, children, father and Bart Kakooza, the man whose phobic tale had precipitated my trip.

Under the murderous regimes of Milton Obote and Idi Amin, Bart Kakooza's and Henry Ford's lifelines to a civil society had been severed. For almost two decades, they could not step out of the fighting, take a breather, replenish emotional resources. They woke up to war outside their window, spent their days with war as their companion and went to bed with war lurking in the shadows. They did this each day without respite, for war allows no weekend breaks, and the days became weeks, months and then years. And through it all, there was not only the job to be done and a living to be made but also a family to care for, children to be raised, nourished and kept safe. Such an existence taxes the hardiest of spirits. War brings not only death and disfigurement, but shortages of food, the collapse of medical services, the disruption of transport, electricity, water, sanitation. It also imbues the traumatized remnants of civil society with a paralyzing ennui. For journalists like Bart and Henry, their work environment had become their home environment, and this blurring of margins, common to all local freelance war journalists, added a new, ominous dimension to the perils faced. Not surprisingly, the consequences of such an existence, both emotional and physical, can be catastrophic.

From the moment I met Henry hobbling along at Entebbe, I was aware of his need to talk and tell me his story. He began en route from the airport into Kampala, even though the hour was late. The following morning I found him waiting for me. The hotel I stayed in was built by the Yugoslav government during the Cold War and later used to billet Idi Amin's thugs. The building, perched on a hill that dominates the landscape, has more recently been resurrected as a Sheraton, and from the windowed dining room you can look down, between gently swaying fronds of Royal Cuban pine, on Kampala's urban sprawl. It was a beautifully clear July morning, and Henry told me the circumstances of his injury.

"In the morning, before I took my children to school," he said, "I told my wife that I was going to the west of the country. Some rebel soldiers had been captured, with their tattered clothing and stained teeth, and I interviewed them. That evening, around ten, I was driven from the army headquarters to a local town. We were told the area had been secured, so I was not expecting trouble. I was sitting in the front seat of an army jeep when suddenly a man appeared out of the dark, pulled open the door, pushed me out and just shot me at close range. I was shot in the stomach and the hip. One of the bullets passed through my hip—it almost took off the neck of the femur—hit part of the pelvis and became embedded in the right buttock.

"I never lost consciousness and lay on the road for about twenty minutes. I only realized my leg was broken when I tried to sit up and the discomfort started. When I touched my trousers, they were all soaked in blood and I could feel some hot stream. Soon our soldiers arrived because they had heard the shots, and I started crying out and saying who I was. 'I'm a native reporter. Please don't kill me. Leave me alone. I'm not a soldier. Don't kill me.' The soldiers recognized me, picked me up, put me in their jeep and that was when the real pain started.

"I was taken into the hospital's examination room at 1:30 a.m. The two doctors on duty were friends of mine, one a family friend and the other had gone to university with me. The hospital, which serves the whole country, had only one theater in operation at the time. My operation took five hours. I would end up having five further operations and staying in hospital for five months. One of the bullets had ruptured the rectum, and I needed a colostomy. Rupturing the rectum caused an infection in part of the shattered femur, an osteomyelitis, and the bone would not heal, so the whole series of operations was designed to remove parts of the infected bone. Eventually the surgeon explained that the head of the femur was getting very little blood and that he was going to cut out this bit. And I asked, 'What do I remain with,' and he said, 'You remain with a leg without a bone.' Of course I believed that could not happen, a limb that is supported only by the flesh. And all this came about because the hospital ward is supposed to accommodate 20 patients but had 150 at that time."

Uganda had only recently returned from the abyss, and the scars are not just to be found in what Henry told me. Kampala, "the hill of antelopes," is a beautiful city, but the crumbling infrastructure presents hurdles for the disabled. Throughout the day Henry chaperoned me, hopping around on his one good leg, his crutches getting in the way of everything, slowing him down, tripping me up, every little task an effort, his infernal sticks interfering with the steering wheel, under the feet of waiters and porters, clattering on the marble floors of the hotel as they slide from the side of his chair, the worn padding and chipped wood attesting to their constant use. Without them, Henry would be helpless, reduced to immobility, unable to leave his house. But I could see that this lifeline to the world was also tormenting him. The most basic of activities had become laborious. Getting in and out of a car requires a new dexterity, polished steps are a source of anxiety, narrow doorways and passageways a constant challenge. Kampala's uneven pavement is an obstacle course that has to be carefully negotiated lest he place his stick in one of the many sidewalk potholes, risking a fall and a whole set of new medical complications.

Henry's outward demeanor—cheerful, even buoyant—was at odds with the dark and morbid content of his thoughts. These spilled out incessantly, an accumulation of eighteen months of hellish misery that he laid before the doctor visiting from the comfort of life in the First World. Henry wasted little time introducing this theme, and he alluded to it often, weaving it into his tale as a way of underscoring his plight: the wealth of Canada versus the poverty of Uganda, the technical expertise of the developed nations versus the bumbling incompetence of the Third World ("There is always bread on the table in the First World"), the difficulties earning money as a freelance journalist in the Third World ("Not like in the developed nations"). The variations were unsettling, which, whether unconsciously or with premeditation, was the desired effect. I could see that in Bart's absence, Henry was using every moment of the day to obliquely solicit my help in his recovery, except he did not come out and state this clearly, preferring a circuitous route, one that embraced harrowing anecdote with physical observation. I could not fault him. A confluence of circumstances presented him with the briefest window of opportunity, the one chance for a young man to heal himself and get back his dignity and self-respect. Perhaps it was pride that prevented him from asking directly for help, or perhaps the elaborate pirouetting was culturally mediated. It mattered not. I was deeply moved by his plight. But the discomfort that I felt stemmed from compassion coupled with a sense of powerlessness. I am a researcher, not a tycoon. I do not have the means to fund this man's medical care, which would entail a visit to South Africa for surgery and a lengthy hospital stay in a private clinic. The best I could do was to bring Henry's story to the attention of the few people who fund my research. Where that would lead was difficult to say.

The irony of Henry's situation is that his life is falling apart at exactly the point when Uganda is beginning to rebuild. He has lost half a femur, and his one leg hangs limp and useless, the muscles shortening by the month. He has no insurance, he cannot earn a decent living, he has a wife and three young children to support, a mortgage, school fees, amenities, rates and taxes to pay. He cannot run and play with his kids, he cannot pick them up, he cannot bathe them as he did before, he cannot tend to his house, he cannot live a decent, fulfilling life. The pressure of it all is suffocating him with worry and guilt, and he is trapped, because there is no money. He is forty years old. What does the future hold for him? What will become of his family? All around him, people, colleagues, family friends, are getting ahead. There are opportunities to be had, but they are passing him by because opportunity does not knock for a cripple. And a cripple is what he has become—that bitter word surfacing time and again in his speech—someone who has let his family down, who cannot provide, who is a burden, a source of worry, not support, a useless appendage, like that flail limb that has come to define in his mind who he really is.

Henry wanted to take me to the National Museum. There was a lull in his story as we went looking for the admission office. The doors to the museum stood ajar, but there was no one about, and the cavernous entrance was devoid of people and furnishings. There was no ticket office, no gift shop, no excited queues of schoolchildren milling about. We wandered in. The exhibition halls were deserted. Everything echoed, our voices, the squelch of my shoes, the clickity-clack of Henry's crutches. We moved along to some dusty display cases; the typed labels behind the glass were yellowing with age, their corners upturned in places. I wondered how much had changed since colonial times, whether the displays predated independence in 1962. A melancholic air hung over the deserted museum. This was not the place to view the beauty, richness and diversity of Ugandan culture. I reminded myself that this country, in Churchill's view, the pearl of Africa, had only recently emerged from a protracted civil war. The university, the museum— these were the institutions that suffered as the military grew fat.

As we got ready to leave, I came across a gap in the drywall and stepped through into a junk-filled room. Standing in the center was a dusty Model T Ford. The sight of the vehicle led Henry to divulge the origins of his name. Family lore has it that Henry's father was born in a Model T, and local custom dictates that propitious events surrounding a birth be incorporated into a person's name. In time, the name Ford was passed on to the next generation. Now Henry has three daughters, spelling the end of the patronymic.

We made our way back to the hotel and sat in a garden, shaded by giant palms. The lawn was immaculately clipped and where it ended, rich soil peeked through beneath the luscious foliage and purple-pink bougainvillea. The temperature was a perfect and unchanging twenty-four degrees Celsius, the breeze warm and without trace of humidity. I remarked to Henry that in Uganda God has his finger on the thermostat, and he smiled gently and said it is good that way because in the past the finger might have been on the trigger. I winced at this reply and fell silent. Henry's eyes were not open to the beauty surrounding him, or if they were, he clearly felt that now was not the time for superficial discussion.

Personal matters were more pressing. He confided that he was worried about his family, particularly his middle daughter.

"It was the two eldest children, whose ages are thirteen and nine years, who were most affected by my shooting," Henry said. "Particularly Tina, the second one. In fact, when I came home from hospital, she would bring me my shoes, always ask me if I wanted something. She could not do enough for me, and when she went off to school, you could see she was not happy about it. While I was in hospital, she wrote a letter. 'Dear Daddy, we are praying so much that you will recover. I also pray that the people who wanted to shoot you also be punished.' My daughter now cannot write a sentence without spelling words in a strange way, and before my shooting she was an A student. And looking back, I remember that when I came out of hospital, this same girl had developed stuttering speech. She could not speak well. It was only after a month or two that she started stabilizing her speech."

Listening to Henry's account of Tina's difficulties, I recognized similarities between her symptoms and those of the war journalist who presented at my hospital with a quasi stroke. The child too had a conversion disorder, her emotional distress finding an outlet in symptoms that resemble neurological dysfunction. What differentiated her from the war journalist was not just her age but also the fact that the stresses she endured were not directly life-threatening. It was her father's narrow escape from death and the resultant family upheaval that became the basis for her anguish, the stammer and jumbled spelling the conduit for her suppressed fears.

My heart went out to this man. Not only did he struggle daily with a useless leg, but the burden was magnified by gnawing guilt, his daughter's failure at school a constant reminder of how he had let his family down. "My children are only in their teens. Why should they suffer?" he asked with quiet desperation. "My father did not make me suffer. My children are now suffering because of me. I'm crippled. I cannot move to places because I am on crutches.

I'm supposed to be their provider, their protector. I'm supposed to be their everything. I go to visit them at school and colleagues look at me as a cripple. So why should I keep looking like this?'"

The last sentence was a direct challenge. But to whom? Me, the doctor from wealthy Canada? His profession that has deserted him? A health care system that has failed him? The answer was probably a combination of all these. Henry reminded me of a modern-day Ahab, but unlike the angry mariner he had focused his bitterness not on exacting revenge but on a fate that had abandoned him. "One of the problems we have in Third World countries," he railed, "is that there exists a very big gap between us and our counterparts, our colleagues in the developed world." He was right, of course, and this is the gist of the matter, for it had been his misfortune to get seriously wounded while working in a profession that makes little money, in a Third World country that lacks the necessary medical expertise to restore his leg.

The shadows lengthened across the lawn. Henry reached for his sticks and hopped onto his one good leg. He would like me to meet his family and offer an opinion on his daughter. Could we get together this evening? He would call for me in an hour. I returned to my hotel room. I had been in the country less than twenty-four hours and felt weighed down by what I had seen and heard. While the empty, echoing halls of the National Museum dampened my spirits, it was Henry's relentless intensity that proved the biggest challenge. He had become my shadow and his predicament was painful to observe. For Henry, there remained a single, last hope. Me. And my discomfort stemmed from the knowledge that I might not be able to help him. I rehearsed what I needed to tell him to disabuse him of the notion that my arrival in the country was his guaranteed salvation.

But whatever speech I prepared would have to wait once I saw Henry and two of his daughters in the foyer. They were the most delightful children, pretty, lively, inquisitive, beautifully turned out in their school uniforms. We made our way downtown to the Grand

Imperial Hotel, where Henry's wife would join us shortly. Twilight is brief on the equator, and the darkened streets of Kampala had emptied by the time we arrived at the old colonial hotel. It was a gloomy place, although there were clues from the faded decor and grand lounge that it has not always been this way. I followed Henry down a dank corridor that led to an outdoor swimming pool surrounded on all sides by tiered hotel rooms. The area was deserted save for a small group drinking off in a corner and a band of musicians who had their amplifiers turned up, the sound reverberating in the emptiness. There was an overpowering smell of chlorine.

It was too noisy to talk there, so we moved to the balcony, where we were soon joined by Charity, Henry's wife. Immediately the couple started discussing Tina, their middle daughter, sitting opposite me. They talked as though she was not present. They were concerned about her school performance because she had to repeat a year. They were upset by her stupidity and complained that shouting at her had not made one bit of difference. They were at their wits' end. What could be wrong with the child? She wasn't like this a few years back.

I was startled by Henry and Charity's attitude. I had assumed they understood that Tina had been traumatized by Henry's shooting. And then I realized, of course, that they had made a connection between the shooting and subsequent emotional distress, but any link between the traumatic event and a symptom like stuttering had eluded them. I interrupted the parents and turned my attention to Tina. She had been sitting at her father's side, impassive, seemingly inured to her parents' harangue, but she livened up immediately and asked about my children, laughed when I told her about the height of the snow in the Canadian winter. Her older sister joined in, and we made easy small talk, about school and singing in the choir and what they did for fun on weekends. There was no sign of stuttering in Tina's speech, and she came across as a lovely, bright, articulate child. I asked the sisters what they would like to be when they grew up, and Lena answered unhesitatingly, a lawyer. Her parents laughed. And Tina, what do you want to be? She hesitated and then quietly replied, a nurse. And why a nurse, Tina? So that I can care for people and help them get better. Henry was incredulous. A nurse! You never told us, Tina! A nurse!

I asked the children to run off and play in the lounge and then explained to Henry and Charity the principles underlying conversion disorder. They gaped. It could not be, said Henry. I assured him it could and quoted the example of the female war journalist. The scales fell from their eyes. I urged them to stop the criticisms. Of course, of course, they agreed. They looked crestfallen.

———

Later that evening Bart arrived at the hotel, straight from the Sudan, covered in a reddish dust, buoyant, vigorous, profusely apologetic for not meeting me at Entebbe. His obvious physical vitality and high spirits were the counterpoint to Henry's labored hops, shuffles and morbid preoccupations. The roles could so easily have been reversed, a quirk of fate setting these two friends and colleagues apart, pulling Henry and family off on a tangent the outcome of which is unclear while leaving Bart to orbit solo in the hostile environs of front-line war reporting. In my many interviews I had come across similar cases of journalists simply being in the wrong place at the wrong time with serious, often catastrophic consequences. But never had the contrast between survivor and victim been more starkly illustrated than with these two friends. And the differences were heightened, given an added emotional valence by the environment in which they lived and worked. Nowhere were the hazards of being a freelance journalist more cruelly exposed than in the Third World, where no amount of scenic beauty or warmth and hospitality could camouflage the fact that a bullet through the hip meant doom.

But in the end, I was in Uganda to answer Bart's dramatic question about his inability to eat meat. A plausible explanation had readily presented itself: bearing witness to the murder of men, women and children, the majority hacked to death with machetes, is likely to unsettle the heartiest of appetites. Now, after meeting with Bart and noting the details of what he experienced and filmed in Rwanda, I partially confirmed my original hypothesis. But I also learned how inadequate my imagination had proved in assembling the collective weight of his war experience.

"I will show you a video of what was happening," Bart told me. "I had a camera with a long zoom so I could see what was actually happening. I witnessed the people being hacked. At one time we went to a place where the rebels had thrown a grenade inside the house, and about twenty people had died in the attack and it was very fresh, happening maybe thirty or forty minutes before. Others were still alive, and the place was littered with pieces of human flesh."

Bart had also reported on events in the Congo, where a civil war had ignited in 1998. "On one occasion there was a firefight going on, and I looked up to see a soldier surrendering," he recalled. "He had put his hands up and then down again as he approached us. And then I could see why he had put his hands down because he was holding his intestines in his hands, and it was terrible. I begged the rebels not to shoot him, and we could see that the bullet had gone right through him. They put him on a truck and took him away. He was still alive, but I think he must have died later on."

While we talked Bart and I were walking along the banks of Lake Victoria while his young son Clive played off to the side. It was a bucolic Sunday. Out on the lake, fishermen cast nets from their dhows. Kampala society had flocked to the waterfront and nearby equestrian center, and my gloomy impressions of the past few days gave way before the abundant signs of a society transforming itself. But shadows from the past were everywhere. I noticed small groups of Asians, returnees of a once-vibrant culture summarily expelled by Idi Amin in the 1970s. Amin himself had had a house close by, and in the bountiful waters of the lake, carp grew to enormous proportions, feeding off the corpses dumped by his henchmen.

I shifted my focus back to what Bart was telling me, for it was Rwanda's recent history that was so troubling to him. "I saw a lot of flesh in Rwanda," he said. "A lot of dead people. Every time I would go to eat meat, I would look at the piece of meat and imagine the stench of some of the rotting bodies. And that would affect me. There were so many pieces of human meat rotting that it really worked on me. I gradually found I could not eat meat any more. When I look at it, it gives me bad ideas. I've tried to brush it out of my mind, but it comes back and my thoughts say, 'Look here. You remember that human flesh you saw rotting? It looked like this.' Recently I was in the eastern part of the Congo, where two tribes were clashing over a little matter and more than five hundred people were killed, just like that, in cold blood. The violence terrified me. You see somebody's kidneys hanging out and they are rotting, and then you go back and they bring you liver in a restaurant. I can't eat it, so you see how it has affected me."

Troubling as the symptoms were for Bart, his difficulties were circumscribed, the phobia well demarcated and exerting little effect on his ability to function as a journalist. It had not spilled over into a more pervasive and generalized anxiety. He is a resourceful man who had simply modified his diet to exclude meat. There were, however, circumstances he could not control, and it was during those moments that his distress, quiescent beneath a regimented lifestyle, reared up and challenged him anew. On his trip through the Sudan, for example, hungry after days of eating very little, he arrived at a village, where a meal was prepared for him. The villagers were poor, but whatever food they had was shared in homage and welcome. In this case, it was meat. This presented an exquisite dilemma for Bart, his phobia at odds with his sense of propriety and his reluctance to offend his hosts. On this occasion he fought his nausea and ate, but there were other times when he was not so strong.

Bart wanted to show me some of his archival material. He had filmed a lot of death in Africa. The offices of Media Plus were housed in the basement of the Nile International Conference Centre, and we gathered there the following morning, Henry in tow. The two small, windowless offices were crowded, and people squeezed past one another as they came and went. In Bart's private office, the press of flesh was no less intense and the close atmosphere was made worse by the loud and excited chatter. There were photographs on the wall, including a series of Bart with President Museveni. Henry and Bart talked at the same time, gesturing excitedly to one particular five-by-seven image pinned loosely to the wall. I moved closer, trying to make out the content. Soldiers were dumping some bodies into a grave, or so it seemed. One of the corpses had been decapitated, and it was this headless figure that they wished me to see. The sight was gruesome; the severed head hung by a string of dark red flesh from the torso. I was startled as much by the image as by its place of prominence. Why would a man with Bart's phobia display an image such as this? I looked up and saw him smiling, and from that smile I learned yet another lesson from this trip to Uganda. Journalists like Bart have seen so much death and mutilation in the course of their work that they have to a large degree become inured to its horrors. I had occasionally come across this hard-boiled attitude when interviewing war journalists in London but until now I had lacked an opportunity to observe it firsthand. "I don't feel emotion when confronted with loads of dead bodies," confided a television cameraman earlier. "I mean, it's just things that have happened. . . . I've had years of watching people getting blown to bits all over the place, and, you know, watching a few get shot in front of your eyes. I suppose the first time it's a bit of a shock. What's irritating, however, and it really freaks me out, are the responses of policemen in England, for example. They see one murder or one dead body and they just have to retire from stress, for the rest of their lives. They take an early pension. I think, 'It's just life, really, isn't it?' I've dealt with that, although my ex-wife might say differently. She thinks I'm a basket case."

This habituation to unspeakable violence seems necessary if journalists are to function in war zones. Without this protective armor, it would be impossible to deflect the emotional fallout of witnessing such depraved behavior and horrible suffering. Yet I am perplexed by an inconsistency. Phobics are, by definition, avoidant in their behavior. The claustrophobic avoids enclosed spaces, the agoraphobic open and public spaces, the arachnophobic spiders and so on. But Bart, whose phobia derives directly from scenes of mutilation and dismemberment, displays the very images he should be avoiding.

The dividing line separating detachment from callousness is a fine one, and journalists must tread carefully. Exactly what Bart's motives were in immediately drawing my attention to the headless corpse were unclear, but I suspected it was a very direct way of challenging my emotional sensibilities and quickly engaging me in the nature of what he had seen and endured on the battlefields of East and Central Africa. I was also aware that no matter how composed his emotional detachment, the man's armor had been breached.

We left Bart's office and went into his editing room. Bart and Henry wanted me to view some of the video material from Rwanda, the Congo and Sudan. A collection of friends, colleagues and hangers-on were introduced, a chair was found for me, center stage, in front of an array of television screens, and the first tape inserted. I was conscious of the others watching me, keenly observing my reactions to what I was about to see. The material was clearly not new to them. What was of greater interest was how the doctor from Canada would react. A picture came into view, of iridescent green hills, heavily cultivated, steeply sloping and disappearing into the clouds. A road wound between the mountains, and in the distance two groups of people walked toward each other. The camera slowly zoomed in on the scene. The group, made up of three or four women stops, hesitant; the second group, comprising half a dozen men, kept moving toward them. They met. There appeared to be some conversation. Suddenly the men raised their hands and started beating the women, who sank to their knees. The camera moved in. What initially appeared to be a beating was much, much worse. The men used machetes and hacked at their victims. The frenzied activity was quickly over, and the men moved off in the direction from which the women had come. A heap of bodies was left lying in the road.

No sound accompanied the film, for the women did not cry out. They did not try to run away or put up a fight. They died quietly, seemingly resigned to their fate, the one brief moment of hesitation on the road their only discernible sign of uncertainty and fear. The image then shifted to a close-up of the massacre, gaping wounds, skin and muscle neatly cleaved down to the bone, crisscross wounds on arms instinctively raised in protection, the partly severed heads and skulls cracked open, the bodies at ungainly angles, huddled together. The continuing absence of any sound imparted a sense of unreality.

There was little chance to gather my thoughts or ask questions, for we moved on to the next scene, a village visited by marauding rogue militiamen not thirty minutes before. If the recently viewed massacre was shocking, the scene in the village beggared belief. At first glance there was nothing unusual to observe: a neatly tended village made up of numerous huts, a well-constructed building with the Red Cross sign denoting a medical clinic. But as the camera got closer the bodies came into view, and they were numerous and everywhere, inside the huts, between the huts, in doorways, out on the paths, between the vegetation. Age was no protection, for some of the victims were a few months old. All bore the imprint of the machete, cleaved flesh and darkening, congealed blood. It was an overwhelming sight, the children and babies who lay in such grotesque, mutilated fashion. I glanced up and observed Henry observing me intently. "You see, Doc? You see what happens here?"

Some villagers survived and were gathered in the clinic. Their wounds were terrible—limbs virtually severed, scalps split to the bone, bathed in blood. They had been numbed into silence. There was no crying, moaning, anger, wail of grief. Even the surviving children had been cowed, shocked beyond vocalizing their distress or crying out in pain. They stared listlessly at the camera, their small bodies a checkerboard of deep, painful wounds.

The film did not end with the massacre. Bart had teamed up with Laurent Kabila's forces as they moved through the jungles of the western Congo, routing the army of Mobutu Sese Seko. En route there was much killing and mutilation, and looting too, for the king of kleptocrats had amassed wealth of staggering proportions. There were astounding scenes attesting to Mobutu's decadence, nowhere more so than in his birthplace, Gbadolite, where the leader had built a series of opulent palaces modeled on those of great European and Oriental dynasties. They stand on a series of hills, surrounded by the squalor of his impoverished, bilked subjects—vast rooms of marble, baths the size of swimming pools, sculpted gardens, extravagant fountains, giant kitchens staffed by French gourmet chefs, gadgetry to open windows and swivel the bed. And most remarkable of all, Bart told me of a life-size sculpture of the mother of the nation cradling the baby Mobutu. The figure had been forged from bronze—all except the penis, that is. Here the leader demanded a metal more precious, no doubt feeling the family jewels deserved special acknowledgment. Gold sated the ego. Faced with such riches, Kabila's forces enthusiastically laid waste to the palaces, Mobutu's genitals an early target.

Compared with the myriad difficulties presented by Henry Ford, Bart's problem was a relatively simple one. He had a phobic disorder of moderate severity that did not affect him unduly. Such a condition is amenable to behavior therapy, and I outlined the principles of graded exposure. Bart listened attentively and readily grasped what needed to be done. To aid him in his treatment, I promised to send him one of the many self-help workbooks that can readily be found in most First World bookstores.

The session over, we left the building, descending a great expanse of stairs. A few yards away, perched on some overhanging masonry, was a vulture. What was this scavenger doing there? Bart told me they were first attracted by the city's abattoirs. Then he stopped and pointed to a large, overgrown field in front of the Uganda International Conference Centre. The name of Idi Amin was evoked yet again. Like Lake Victoria, the field had become a dumping ground for those killed. The vultures, like the carp, grew fat. In time, the killing stopped. But the vultures remained, adapting to life in the midst of a million living people.

6

WAR, WOMEN, WIVES AND WIDOWS

*[War creates] a barrier of indescribable experience
between men and the women they loved. Quite early I
realized the possibility of a permanent impediment to
understanding.*

— VERA BRITTAIN

In October 2001, just before the start of the American
bombing in Afghanistan, a female journalist from the
Express newspaper in the United Kingdom donned a
full burka, hired two local stringers and slipped across the Pakistan border astride a donkey. Beneath the billowing folds of her
disguise, she carried a camera and her notebook. Yvonne Ridley
was intent on viewing militant Islamic fundamentalism at first
hand. In this she succeeded, although the manner in which she
came by her story was unplanned and hardly imaginable. Her
undoing resulted entirely from the capriciousness of her donkey.

"I had been in Afghanistan for two days, undercover, and I was
heading back to the Pakistan border, about twenty minutes away,
when the beast bolted," she told me during an interview at the BBC

television studios in White City, London. "As I careered past some Taliban, my camera swung into view. When the soldier pulled me off the donkey and took my camera, everything just shut down. I went totally numb. I was without emotion. And it was as if I was watching myself. It was quite weird. I felt as though I was observing the Taliban and this other woman who was me, and I could hear my own voice, in a disconnected way, talking to them and explaining I was English, not American. I dipped in and out of that type of feeling over the course of the ten days I was in captivity."

What Ridley described to me is, in psychiatric parlance, an account of dissociation, a splitting-off of part of a person's mental faculties as a response to significant stress. Taken to its most florid manifestation, dissociation can cause a person to have a complete out-of-body experience, in which she looks down on herself as a physically separate person. Lesser variants are more common. When Yvonne Ridley was defrocked by the Taliban, she experienced one such symptom. Called depersonalization, it refers to the sensation of being cut off from an aspect of self, be it the voice, actions, or parts of the body.

In Ridley's case, her dissociative experiences would wax and wane over the course of her ten-day ordeal. During the drive to a holding cell in Jalalabad, she recalled that "they suddenly stopped the car, and the soldier got out and placed me on this raised piece of ground. So I am standing there, and the burka is off, and these men started gathering around, staring at me, getting closer and closer, and I just thought I was about to be stoned. They say your life flashes by when you're going to die, but all I could think of was, I hope that when they start stoning me, the first one knocks me out. What sort of pain am I going to feel? Will my mom and dad ever find out? Will they have to identify my body? What state will my body be in? Will Daisy, my daughter, ever find out? It's just a horrible way to die. And I am looking at these people getting closer and closer, and I can't even beg for mercy because that's just going to make everything worse. This is a barbaric regime. So I just stood there and the Taliban soldier flagged down a car. He was looking for a woman to search me. I was so relieved that I was not going to be stoned, but this quickly gave way to anger that these bastards had terrified the life out of me. So I turned around and went to rip my dress as if to say, I'm not carrying anything. I had trousers on and lifted up my dress and the men just went, 'Aaagh!' and started running in the other direction. Everything suddenly spun from high drama to high farce."

From Jalalabad, Ridley was transferred to a prison in Kabul. Her labile behavior persisted as she swung between quiet periods of obedience and episodes of uncontrollable rage and frustration. The one constant was fear. "I would have repeated episodes where I would do something and say something and I'm thinking, Where the hell is this coming from? One day when I was up in Kabul prison, the Taliban came to see me and said, 'We're going to ask you some more questions.' I was in the courtyard at this point and I just said, 'I'm finished with questions. I'm not going to answer any more of your questions. Just go away.' They said, 'We are very concerned. You're not eating, you're our guest, you're like a sister.' I just exploded and I said, 'I'm not your sister, I don't have any brothers, and if I had brothers like you I'd disown them.' And I also said, 'I'm not your guest, I can't walk out of here. You've locked me in this horrible prison. You know you judge civilization by the quality of its prisons. Well, let me tell you, you people are primitive.' And I ended the conversation by saying, 'Now get out of my sight,' and I went and spat at them and walked back into my cell. And I was trembling like a leaf, really shaking, and the Christian Aid workers who were there said, 'Yvonne, you were very robust.' And I said, 'I've gone too far and I'm very, very scared.' I was standing there just trembling. I think it was the first time I'd actually trembled, and my mouth had gone very dry, I remember that. One female came in and translated for me. She said, 'You are going to be flogged because you cannot speak to high people like that.' Again, I just seemed to be out of my body, watching me. I just couldn't believe the crap that I came out with. I just said, 'Well, if I am flogged and I feel pain, then I will know that I am still alive.' And I'm thinking, Where is this shit coming from?'"

Ridley's story is remarkable on many levels. A foreign woman journalist had crossed the hostile border of a fundamentalist Islamic state that treats her sex harshly. She had no documentation, was in disguise, and war between her country and this state was imminent. Soon, she was captured, but rather than show contrition, she verbally insulted her captors and spat in the faces of those who would decide her fate. History is littered with the corpses of people who have done far less to irritate the sensitivities of totalitarian regimes. As our interview progresses I try to make sense of Ridley's volatile behavior. Is this woman journalist courageous, feisty and spirited in standing up for herself, or did she show foolhardy arrogance, ignorance and appalling insensitivity? What makes her reactions to her Taliban captors so surprising is that Yvonne Ridley comes across as a pleasant, open and friendly woman in interview. There is a vulnerability to her, with none of the hard-edged arrogance she displayed while in captivity. Indeed, even Ridley herself was stunned by her behavior and genuinely perplexed by her inability to control it. Such was her fear at times that any conscious resolve was swamped by emotion, rendering her actions erratic and potentially self-injurious. This intermittently fevered state of arousal triggered discrete dissociative episodes, alarming in themselves because of their foreign, dysphoric and disconnected quality. "I just seemed to be out of my body, watching myself. Where is this shit coming from?" asked Ridley incredulously. To which the answer is, from dissociation, induced by fear, anxiety, uncertainty, helplessness. Her belated appreciation of the potentially deleterious consequences of her actions further heightened her anxiety, thereby perpetuating, if not magnifying, her distress. More erratic behavior followed. This downward spiral, in which one negative emotion fed off another, ended only with her release a few days after the Americans began bombing Afghanistan.

———

Dissociative phenomena are not unusual following traumatic experiences. Other journalists reported them too, but unlike Yvonne Ridley's account, their episodes were non-repetitive and brief. Furthermore, they occasionally manifested away from zones of conflict. My interview with Janine di Giovanni of the *Times* illustrates these points well. We met on a wet and chilly summer's day in a London office overlooking Hyde Park. Slanting sheets of rain smacked against the window, blurring the greenery outside, and sounds of traffic drifted up from the street below. At first, the conversation was dominated by events in Bosnia and her description of life under siege in Sarajevo. At one point in her narrative, she fell silent, took a sip of her coffee and lay back on the settee, eyes closed. I waited silently for her thoughts to coalesce, avoiding the temptation to break the stillness with another question or observation. When di Giovanni resumed talking she had switched continents and moved on to Africa and the civil war in Sierra Leone. Two months back, not far from the capital, Freetown, in a nondescript section of bushveld known as Rogberri Junction, her colleagues Kurt Schork and Miguel Gil Moreno were ambushed and killed. She too had traveled that area.

"I had just gotten back from Sierra Leone, where I had been for a month," she recalled. "I had become used to seeing amputees. They are everywhere in that sad society, and they have this kind of freaky thing they do with the stumps of their severed limbs, waving them about. I had flown back to Paris, and the day after I arrived I found out that my friends had been killed. I was walking down this street and had this weird hallucination, which I have never had before. It was a very crowded street, and all these people coming toward me were amputees. I had to tell myself, Hold on, you're in Paris now, you're in Paris, it's fine. It's okay. And then, just as suddenly, they were gone."

This transient, intense perceptual disturbance occurs with full insight—that is, an appreciation by the journalist that something is amiss. When reality briefly distorts, the experience is termed derealization. Di Giovanni's derealization and Ridley's depersonalization are both variants of dissociation that may occur in response to overwhelming anxiety-provoking events. The fact that the first two cases I encountered were in women suggested, albeit tentatively, that male and female war journalists differed in the nature and extent of their psychopathology. This in itself would not be unexpected, for a consistent medical finding in the general population is that women are twice as likely as men to experience conditions such as post-traumatic stress disorder, major depression and anxiety disorders. Reasons for this vary from differences in hormonal and biochemical makeup to a greater willingness on the part of females to discuss feelings and emotions.

With these facts in mind, I reanalyzed the data comparing the responses of the 110 male war journalists with their 30 female counterparts. The most immediate observation was the disparity in numbers. There were almost three male journalists for every female. This contrast was most obvious in the area of stills photography, where only two photographers were female. It was, however, with respect to their psychological profile that results were most striking, for no differences were present on any measure of psychopathology. Female journalists were no more depressed, anxious, somatically preoccupied, socially dysfunctional or suicidal, in other words, than male journalists. Nor did they appear any more prone to the re-experiencing, avoidant or arousal symptoms of PTSD. And although my data did not unearth further cases of dissociation, I did hear of other examples expressed by male journalists who were not part of my study. None was more dramatic and evocative than the account given by the BBC's Anthony Massey, who had covered the Balkan wars. He related an episode during which, on a London street and in broad daylight, the building in front of him transformed into the facade of a Sarajevo hotel and slowly began disintegrating under bombardment. Like the visual perturbation that had unsettled Janine di Giovanni, the episode was very brief and insight was retained.

This failure to identify more psychological difficulties in females suggested a possible demographic divide between the genders, but here the results once again confounded expectations. The average age of the female war journalists (thirty-nine years) matched that of the males, and both groups had been working in zones of conflict for approximately fifteen years, so there was no evidence that females had reported fewer symptoms because they had less exposure to danger and conflict. The one area where there was a gender difference was the marital data: only 24 percent of the female journalists were married compared with 52 percent of their male counterparts.

If married female war journalists are a minority, those with children are even rarer. Only three of the thirty women in my study had children, and in each case, they had only one child apiece. Yvonne Ridley was one. At some point in her interview with me she began crying and seemed embarrassed by the display of emotion. "This is the first time I have wobbled when I've been out of the house," she confessed. The main source of her distress was not what had occurred in Afghanistan but rather the criticism she faced from many of her peers on her return home. She was accused of both endangering the safety of her two local stringers and abrogating her responsibilities as the mother of an eleven-year-old daughter. The latter was particularly hurtful and resented, and it raises the question whether the battlefields of war are uneven from a gender perspective. When aspersions are cast on the maternal competency of female war journalists while the many fathers, most with more than one child, are allowed to escape the same moral scrutiny, the charge of sexism becomes hard to refute. All the women I interviewed saw it as the perpetuation of a stereotype of the mother as the parent who is most responsible for the upbringing of a child. This left the dads free to go off to the office, which in this profession happened to be the caves of Tora Bora or the ruins of Kandahar. Female war journalists, in choosing voluntarily, willingly, hungrily to enter zones of conflict, shatter the mold of compliant domesticity. And yet, despite their fierce determination to succeed in the male-dominated domain of war, described to me by Maggie O'Kane as "boys in sleeveless jackets talking about incoming and outgoing," most women chose non-front-line assignments or gave up war journalism altogether when they had children. The exceptions, unlike the men, are a very small minority.

For those few mothers working in far-off zones of conflict, weighing the risks of the job against their commitment as parents presented uncomfortable choices. How they resolved these competing agendas was a question I put to O'Kane, the mother of a young son, when we met on a blustery cold morning at a café in north London. She cited the conflict in East Timor, which she did not cover, as an example of the various forces that would inform her decision making. She said it was the behavior of the *Sunday Times* reporter Marie Colvin that she admired most, for Colvin had refused to join the mass evacuation during the Indonesian militia's reign of terror. "She stayed when it was really important," O'Kane told me. "Everyone, including the United Nations, was preparing to abandon the East Timorese. The UN had done that before in Srebrenica, you know. And they were embarrassed by this one woman who was broadcasting relentlessly. 'I'm surrounded by women and children. The younger children are crying. The militiamen are outside.' That kind of stuff, you know. There were five hundred journalists hanging around in Darwin. All of them had cleared off too. Hundreds of journalists had cleared out because someone had a stone thrown at them, or got their leg broken, or got shot. The local people really needed us then. They had had a democratic election. They had put their faith in the UN and their courage too. And these journalists had all fucked off, basically. So

I ask myself, Would I have stayed in East Timor if I'd been with Marie?" O'Kane grew silent, pondering her own challenge. She took a long swig from her early-morning Coca-Cola, before resuming more hesitantly. "I think if I had been with Marie, I probably would have stayed, because I would have taken my courage from her. And then I would have had this dilemma, you know. I'm a mother. What am I going to do? Maybe that thought would have made me want to leave. And then I would have looked around me and seen all the mothers with their children. The only thing that protected them was the press. I'm not being heroic about this, but I'd like somehow to be useful."

Personal courage aside, the reality is that gender does, on occasion, become an issue. For one thing, women are more vulnerable to sexual assault in war zones where civil society has crumbled and lawlessness often prevails. Genocide in Bosnia and Rwanda are just two recent examples of how, as part of the organized terror, the female population was systematically and methodically brutalized.

I asked all the female journalists I interviewed how much of a threat sexual assault was. While all acknowledged it was a concern, only one had ever been directly threatened with rape. Conversely, many female war journalists reported instances of male combatants going out of their way to be protective. One photographer told me, "On a number of occasions some of the soldiers wouldn't let me go into a conflict zone. They were motivated out of a sense of protection. At times they actually held me back physically from going. And I refused to submit to this restriction. I think they just felt it was their duty as men within that society, particularly in Bosnia. They would just not allow women to go into situations that were potentially hazardous, be it sexually or physically. And while I could understand that, I could not agree with it. Women do not have a monopoly on reporting stories of civilian issues, casualties, struggles, nor do men have a monopoly on access to the combatants."

At times, when a woman was caught in a hazardous situation, the fear of a summary execution was so real that it superseded any concerns about rape. One female reporter told me of a harrowing episode that took place in Kosovo at the start of the bombing campaign. "I just wandered across the border and was picked up by Serb paramilitary," she recalled. "I was with two male French journalists, and the soldiers marched us off into the woods and basically staged a mock execution. They kept us for about an hour and a half. They were drunk. And then they received some news, which we later found out was the capture of an American pilot, and they decided to let us go. I guess they did not need captives any more. Afterward, the French cameramen said they were more afraid for me because they thought I was going to be raped. In truth, it had not crossed my mind. I thought they were going to kill us. A bullet in the back of the head. But not rape."

She went on to say, "The risks are greater in Africa. In places like Sierra Leone, for example, where there are these young soldiers, children often, high on drugs. And then there is the aspect of a crowd-driven war. You are in a crowd, suddenly some incident happens, they go wild and chaos happens very quickly. It is more savagely unpredictable. There is something very primitive about that type of reaction in Africa. I do think that Serb militia, as much as they might be brutal, would not even contemplate raping a journalist. Chechens would probably do it. But a bunch of African kids, stoned—what does the Geneva Convention mean to them?"

The one female journalist I interviewed who had been threatened with rape was on assignment in Africa, where she was taken hostage briefly by some rogue militiamen. Unlike her female colleagues who had never been exposed directly to such threats, this journalist did not have to draw on conjecture or her imagination when I asked for her views. Her ordeal took place when she had just completed an assignment in Southern Africa and was ready to return home. "There were seven guys waiting for me at the international airport," she told me. "They knew I was leaving that day. They did not introduce themselves. They had guns and a Motorola. They were quite young and they said, 'You come with us.'

They just grabbed me and I said no. I started screaming at the top of my voice, and there was a Lufthansa crew there—you know, the stewards—and I shouted, 'Somebody help me,' because I knew something bad was going to happen, but nobody did. I was screaming my head off. I felt like a madwoman in this international airport, stewards not doing anything. The soldiers took me into this room downstairs and went through my bag, took my tapes and said, 'You're an enemy of the people. You are a bad woman.' They started to undress me, and I thought I was going to be raped."

The timely intervention of a military attaché who had witnessed the abduction stopped the assault from going any further, but it had been a close call and it left a lingering, troubling aftermath. "Even now, eight months later, when I see black men, they piss me off. I can't stand the smell of them. And I become fearful, because they have a certain smell, particularly in Africa, where it is so hot and humid. I was never this way before."

An episode like this was the exception, however. More common was the kind of bumbling, fumbling attempts described by Yvonne Ridley after her capture. En route to Jalalabad in a car, she was set upon by one of her guards. "This man, who was not Taliban, started touching me, groping me. I told him to stop and he didn't, so I winded him. A Taliban soldier in front had seen part of this, and he kicked the groper out the car."

At times, the threat comes not from militiamen, combatants or drunk soldiers but instead from a colleague, as one camerawoman recalled. "I generally work on my own, but on one of my trips to Pakistan and Afghanistan to get an interview with the one-eyed Mullah Omar, leader of the Taliban, I needed the help of a local journalist. He worked for one of the main newspapers on the northern frontier that was published in English and Urdu. So we met up in Pakistan and went out for some food before going back to his office, where we shared a joint of hash. And while smoking, he asked me, 'What is love like?' One minute we are talking about the Taliban and the next, 'Tell me what love is like.' And I said,

'Well, why are you asking? You're married, you have kids—aren't you in love with your wife?' 'No, she's my first cousin.' I said, 'You're an educated guy. Why did you marry your first cousin?' He said, 'Tribal society. I had to.' And then he pounced on me. He was a pretty big guy, but luckily I am fairly strong."

These accounts of narrow sexual escapes should not be misconstrued as evidence that female war journalists are under unusually constant siege from predatory males. Even in civil society, sexual harassment is common across all social strata, sparing no occupation. According to a University of Maryland study 60 percent of the women accredited to the Capitol press gallery in Washington reported that they had been sexually harassed. A different study of over ten thousand female employees of the federal government in the United States revealed that one-third had experienced lewd sexual remarks, a quarter had been sexually touched, one in seven had been pressured for dates, one in ten had been pressed for sexual favors and one hundred women had been sexually assaulted or raped. As such, the surprising fact to emerge from the interviews with the women war journalists is not that some have been propositioned, fondled and sexually threatened but that it occurs relatively infrequently. A plausible explanation for this may be the subjective nature of what constitutes sexual badgering. Conflict-hardened war journalists will have a different threshold than civil servants for perceiving danger, be it physical or sexual. At the same time, political correctness in war zones will never assume the Inquisition-like fervor it arouses in federal and corporate offices. What is also singular about the relative lack of sexual threat reported by female war journalists is that it stands in marked contrast to the gross violations often perpetrated on the female civilian population in zones of conflict.

Still, the women journalists I interviewed were undeniably conscious of the dangers they face, even if they were reluctant to concede that their gender confers additional risk. While the infrequency of the assaults may assuage fears and embolden commitment, their psychological defenses are also not hard to detect. "If you are afraid of everything, you wouldn't do it," Janine di Giovanni told me. "If you are going to analyze all these things, forget it. It's like jumping into a swimming pool. If you are going to think how cold it will be, you will never do it. You can't think too much."

———

My interviews did show that female war journalists had some unique characteristics. They differ from the general female population by remaining single into their late thirties and forties and showing a striking resilience to the emotional consequences of trauma. They generally refute the notion that they are particularly vulnerable to sexual assault, and they deny this potential hazard has ever been a deterrent to their pursuing work in the zones of conflict. Their propensity for high risk-taking appears similar to that of their male colleagues, which yet again flies in the face of gender data in general. They also hold that their behavior in war zones, as women and mothers, should not be judged by a set of rules different from those applied to male journalists, especially those who are fathers too.

My data did, however, reveal one area where women journalists may be especially vulnerable to psychological distress. In two of the three mothers I interviewed, childbirth was the catalyst for the recrudescence of repressed traumatic memories. Before describing the details of the two cases, I must point out that the criteria for post-traumatic stress disorder make allowances for a delayed onset of symptoms. The phenomenology of the disorder remains the same—which means some re-experiencing, avoidance and physiological arousal symptoms must be present—but in this instance their onset is delayed by at least six months from the time of exposure to the trauma. The woman whom I interviewed in New York on a late winter's evening had a *forme fruste* (partial form) of PTSD—namely, the presence of prominent re-experiencing symptoms accompanied by some physiological arousal—but she lacked avoidance features. What made her presentation unusual was the delayed onset of intrusive recollections, for they had begun one year after she stopped work as a war journalist.

Her career over the preceding decade had been stellar. Very much part of that inner sanctum of veteran, committed war journalists who regarded their work as a mission, she had, like all of them, come close to getting killed. Her response to a landmine incident demonstrates her psychological resilience to life-threatening events. "It was pretty bad," she recalled. "We were in an armored car, otherwise we would have been blown to bits, and I was in hospital several weeks. I had severe damage in both knees and ankles and this wound in the face. There was also some internal bleeding, but it absolutely did not dent my resolve or confidence." Such was her determination to witness events firsthand that her editor, while acknowledging the quality of her work, urged greater caution. Throughout an intense ten-year period in some of the world's most dangerous places, she had never developed PTSD, depression or enduring psychological distress. And when one day she realized, to her dismay, that a missed scoop had become more upsetting to her than the misery of the countless victims who made up the content of the story, she walked away from her profession.

After leaving conflict journalism, this woman could have been forgiven for thinking she had survived psychologically the horrors she had witnessed. After all, they had never bothered her while she was working, and with imminent dangers now largely behind her, the probability of some tardive psychological decompensation must have been considered remote. She soon became pregnant, and two days after the birth, everything changed. "I started having, and still have to a lesser degree, intrusive memories of very violent events," she confessed. "They just flash into my consciousness. People getting killed. They are very vivid recollections. Of course, after you give birth you realize that in very simplistic terms, everyone that you ever photographed grieving over someone they lost had loved their kid as much as you love your baby. Having a child promotes a higher degree of empathy with the things that we have been covering. So I'd have flashbacks that were extraordinarily vivid. I'll give you an example. One of them was an image of a woman in Bosnia crying over the grave of her second son. She had lost both her sons in the Bosnian war within months of each other. She was just crying inconsolably over the grave. These were the kinds of things that came to me. Later on I started to have intrusive thoughts and images of people doing something violent to my child. Because I've seen people being shot and murdered in front of me, and witnessed the aftermath of such outrages perpetrated on people of all ages, I often have these kinds of things flash into my mind."

This journalist offers a plausible psychological explanation for the delayed onset of PTSD-type symptoms. Becoming a parent and bonding intensely with your newborn awakens strong protective instincts. It also sensitizes you to the grief of those who have lost children in conflict. To this may be added a different but complementary interpretation: that while working as a war journalist she dealt with emotionally painful events she had witnessed by successfully repressing them. The birth of her own child activated her unconscious, awakening images that were forgotten but not quiescent. These psychodynamic theories should also be viewed in their proper biochemical and hormonal context, for the postpartum period is one of rapid and extensive physiological change. It may precipitate fluctuations in mood ranging from the common, transient and minor postpartum "blues" to more serious and disabling episodes of depression or mania. Although in the journalist in question it was not depression that appeared but one aspect of PTSD, the pathogenesis of the symptoms should nevertheless be considered similar.

A second case, with overlapping features, adds weight to this conclusion. Mixing fragments of autobiography with events witnessed as a war reporter, Maggie O'Kane recalled that "in all my years of foreign reporting, feeling the pop of a bullet beside my ear in Timor or lying under a tree trunk in Chechnya looking up at the iron belly of a Russian gunship, nothing compares to the terror of feeling someone is going to hurt your baby."

An article she wrote for the *Guardian* titled "I Feel the Madness More" addresses head-on the emotional conflict between her years as a war reporter and subsequent motherhood. "About a month after my son, Billy, was born I took a walk on London's Hampstead Heath," she recounted. "We were alone. Me, an ecstatic mother in my new camel-hair Christmas coat and a small boy in an old-fashioned bouncy pram his grandmother had sent from Glasgow." It was then that O'Kane noticed a stranger emerge from the wood. "A man with his shoulders rounded up toward his ears" is how she remembered him. "He had a black V-neck pullover. No shirt. He wasn't wearing a coat. He walked past us. He never looked up. I kept walking along the muddy path, never changing my pace, never turning my head to see where the man with no eyes was. I saw a bend ahead and turned it. I yanked Billy's pram behind a tree and watched the man in the black sweater. Through what was left of the winter leaves, I saw him stop. His head up now like a gun dog, scanning, turning, then creeping after us. Slow, deliberate, alert, I pulled Billy's pram tight. I heard a voice rasping in my head. I was rehearsing a primeval scream and a message for the man who was coming for my baby. My legs were weak. But I felt a dazzling strength in my body that was completely new to me. I knew that if he touched my child, I would rip his head off with my teeth. For the first time in my life I understood real terror at being unable to protect my child."

The shabby stranger did not attack her. He approached to within ten feet and then mysteriously stopped before turning away. Was he a stalker? Was he planning on harming her newborn son? The reader is left unclear on these points. No such doubts for Maggie O'Kane. Her fevered account of events provides ample proof of her terror. What is significant about this story is not so much the intent of the stranger but her reaction to his odd behavior. The magnitude of her fear is crystallized by a juxtaposition of what occurred on the heath with memories culled from her decade as a war journalist. She describes a visit to Kosovo, in the wake of German NATO troops. "Suva Reka, about twenty miles from our base, was a small town on the road to somewhere else. But for Vjolica Berisha it was the place where she was born, grew up, married and became the mother of three children. In the burned-out shopping precinct past the Beni Tours travel shop, there is a coffee shop with blue bar stools. Here she saw her children murdered. In my mind I still have a picture of the woman trying to hide her toddler between her legs, then feeling the bullet thud into his body." O'Kane managed to find Vjolica Berisha and interview her in a sunny garden in Kosovo. Fifty-three people, mostly women and children from the Berisha family, had died in the attack on the coffee shop. Among the dead were her sister Shyreta's four children. "Motherhood," wrote O'Kane, "had changed the way I would look at war forever."

She gave another example of this new outlook, this time from Cambodia. "In [the] S21 Prison, where the Pol Pot regime executed the higher cadres and their children, the condemned were photographed before execution. Staring out from the wall of the prison museum that still smelt of their blood was a young woman with her six-month-old baby stretched out on the metal bed beside her. She had number 320 pinned to her collar and she looked into the camera with what seemed like powerless acceptance of what was going to happen to her and her baby. Upstairs, somewhere in the dusty archives, were the folders of the condemned. I spent four days searching for something about her. It was an obsession. I was driven through file after dusty file, maddened by the look on her face and by her naked child beside her on the iron frame of the prison bed. I was trying to imagine her mind knowing that, in a day or two, someone would take her baby from her and smash his head open on the trees of the killing fields outside Pnom Penh. They never wasted bullets on children." O'Kane was not yet finished picking at the raw scab of memory, for there is a third harrowing account of loss, one that unfolded in the leukemia ward of the Saddam Hussein Children's Hospital in Baghdad. "I felt the same madness. The figures of two parents stooped over their thirteen-year-old son who would die tomorrow. The drugs he needed were forbidden under sanctions. Imagine watching your child die because some politicians in France, Britain and the U.S. can't think of a better way of getting rid of Saddam. I had sometimes felt anger in my previous trips to Baghdad, but after Billy it was different."

All these horrors have as a central theme parents mourning the loss of a child or children. Each one of these memories assumes an added poignancy for Maggie O'Kane following the birth of her son. Although she is conscious of not equating her narrow escape on Hampstead Heath with the grievous losses of war, she acknowledges that it took becoming a mother and a perceived threat to her own infant before she could begin to understand the depth of anguish she observed in those parents.

O'Kane was four weeks postpartum when she took that frightening walk on a winter's day in north London. Like her colleague, who within days of giving birth began experiencing violent intrusive memories, she too had repressed emotionally troubling images from her time spent reporting war. For each of these women, childbirth was the key that involuntarily unlocked her unconscious. It did not deter Maggie O'Kane from returning to war, but she did so with a heightened sensitivity. Her meeting with Vjolica Berisha took place after the birth of Billy, and it was as a mother that she reacted to the magnitude of Vjolica's loss. "That is the image that haunts me most from ten years on the job," she wrote, "a mother clinging for those last seconds to the body of her two-year-old child. The agony of watching your child die and not being able to protect it."

These two examples are reminders that despite the unusual and distinct profile of women war journalists, there is one area where male and female war journalists diverge, where the women journalists' behavioral responses revert to the mean, coming closer to the typical profile associated with women in the general population. For whether a woman is a librarian or a war journalist, her gender theoretically confers on her a heightened vulnerability to developing psychological symptoms in the days and weeks following childbirth. A final, very personal recollection from O'Kane's *Guardian* article once again illustrates the connection, although in this case it was her own miscarriage that provided the impetus for the return of traumatic memories. She had been pregnant while in Kosovo recording details of the Berisha family's tragedy. "It was a month later, on holiday in Italy, before I knew that the foetus was dead and had waited to miscarry," recalled O'Kane. "In the wonderful hospital near Florence, a fat cheerful gynecologist scanned my then flabby belly: 'It's all gone,' she said, congratulating me on the thorough job my body had done getting rid of the foetus. My husband, standing in the corner of the surgery with Billy in his arms, had tears in his eyes; I felt very little. I can't remember if it was at that moment, or during the long night that my body was rejecting the foetus, that I thought of Shyreta and her four dead children, of those final seconds when she held the body of the smallest one."

My investigation of female journalists and their experiences with childbirth led me to wonder how the partners of war journalists in general were faring emotionally. The few times I had met spouses or former spouses, they had hinted at a Pandora's box of fear, frustration and discord. I therefore wanted to expand my study to include them, and I soon got the chance. CNN and the BBC were prepared to fund a new research protocol.

Using the 140 war journalists from the first study, I contacted a sample of partners scattered over three continents. They were given the study's Internet address and asked to fill out basic demographic data and complete the same questionnaires. By essentially duplicating the original methodology, I would be able to make statistical comparisons between two groups. Sample size was set at thirty subjects, which represented approximately half the total number of married war journalists. The spousal group was predominantly female. This was anticipated, given that only seven of the journalists who were married or cohabiting were female.

The questionnaires showed that war journalists and their spouses had similar scores for depression and psychological distress but not PTSD. This was an important observation because the original study had already established elevated levels of psychopathology in war journalists. The new data extended this finding to their spouses and partners by demonstrating unequivocal signs of similar emotional difficulties, PTSD apart. In other words, evidence of increased psychological distress in the war journalists, be it depression, anxiety, social dysfunction or various combinations of these signs and symptoms, was associated with depression in their partners. Association does not, however, equate with causality, and as such, the data preclude establishing the direction of this relationship. It may well be that the low mood in some spouses is secondary to the emotional dysfunction in their journalist partner, but until this question is directly addressed with a different methodology, such conclusions remain premature.

Informative as these initial results were, I wanted to get between the questions and flesh out more personal and detailed responses from spouses. What was it like to be married to someone who worked in such a hazardous profession? Did they ever adjust to their loved one's jetting off, at short notice, into a war zone? What effects did their partner's peripatetic existence have on their relationship, social contacts, children? What had first attracted them to their partner? Did they know they were marrying a person wedded by temperament to risk taking? A blank text box was placed at the end of the questionnaires to record the spouses' responses.

Before we get into details of the replies, two cautionary points need emphasis. The first is that while male partners of war journalists completed the questionnaires, none supplied anecdotal accounts of what it was like to be married to a female war journalist. The second point is that only one-quarter of the female partners who completed the study used the text box for describing their feelings in greater detail. As such, the views expressed probably do not reflect a consensus opinion. It is quite possible there are wives and husbands who are fully accepting of what their war journalist partners do and are not unduly distressed by the nature of their relationships. If so, I did not hear from them. Similarly, none of the female respondents spontaneously praised an uxorious husband. The open-ended text box may therefore have selectively tapped into a wellspring of spousal frustration, hurt and anxiety. It is with this limitation in mind that the comments I received should be viewed.

All spouses spoke of difficulties in their relationships, and all but one expressed little enthusiasm for the profession of war journalism. In tones of anger, hostility, bitterness and, for some, sadness and resignation, the replies were a litany of complaints directed against the partners. Replies ranged from the disillusioned ("I think the common answer to spouse or partner reaction might be divorce") to the cynical ("One of the constants in this game is that relationships tend not to last very long, which in turn means it's sometimes easier not to have them at all") to the apologetic ("I got a message from my husband about your research on how journalists who cover conflict zones deal psychologically with the stresses of the work and what effects it may have on their partners. I would like to help you, but I do not qualify any more as we are getting divorced. My husband has a new partner and might be able to put you in touch with her"). No signs here of that almost transcendental buzz of excitement experienced by the journalists themselves as they head off to yet another war. In their wake comes a house to run, kids to look after, perhaps a career on hold, a limited family budget to get by on and the challenge of maintaining a veneer of domestic tranquillity in the face of a constant undercurrent of anxiety and worry. Spouses spoke of the impossibility of planning social arrangements in advance, precipitate departures, the abdication of family responsibilities, the difficulties of staying in contact because of poor communication and the struggles of children either confused by a father's prolonged absences or overexcited on his return. "It is very difficult watching the pain of children whose birthdays and precious rites of passage have been ignored, forgotten or overlooked," bemoaned one respondent.

Even the response from the one more upbeat spouse was tinged with a multiplicity of worries and a resigned sense that she had been relegated to a supporting role. She wrote, "Partners of war journalists must be independent, forgiving, mature, willing to sacrifice, feel that he or she is contributing to their spouse's ability to perform an important job, stable enough to be both the father and the mother when necessary, willing to take risks (even though we may not like it), accepting of people's differences and assets, non-egoistic (there isn't usually room for two huge egos in a long-term relationship) and feel respected by their spouse for the role they play." The sentence reads at first like a checklist of attributes that a partner of a war journalist must have in order to sustain the relationship. However, a closer inspection reveals that her last point is not something she can give. Inadvertently, she has interpolated one thing she asks in return: respect.

Notwithstanding these attributes, there's no guarantee her anxieties are kept at bay. She muses, "I wonder how many spouses of war journalists you'll find out there? Most journalists cannot maintain a long-term relationship, for many reasons. I think I have been able to cope because I met my husband very young, was willing to sacrifice many things for our relationship to work, have a strong, stable family background and am able to parent without a partner. You need all this to deal with the stress of 'security' (money, insurance, savings, retirement, etc.). But the biggest issue for people like me is confidence in your spouse to make the correct and safe decisions—and also that your partner will remain sexually faithful. That seems to have been the breaking point for many couples that I know. Matter of fact, we are the only long-term couple still together that I personally know about (that is, where the spouse is not also a journalist)."

Before signing off, she returns yet again to the issue of what she has given up for her husband. "Time away from home is one thing, but time spent when they are at home is another. My husband works almost constantly when he is here. The only down time we have is when we go off on a holiday. Even then he is still constantly being contacted for work. During our last family trip the agency wanted him to leave for Israel. This time he said no. I don't get angry about this kind of life. It is just the way it is. As for the children, they don't know any other kind of father and accept it. That basically is why I don't work—so that at least one parent is there for them."

As we saw earlier, many war journalists experience difficulties adjusting on their return home from a war zone. They're often left alienated by an ordered civil society replete with domestic chores and humdrum routine. The negative effects of a difficult readjustment all too often spill over into relationships and may disturb a family milieu that has already been unsettled by a hurried departure. "Partners often feel very stressed that their spouses are in such danger," one wife explained. "Family life can be difficult when the journalist comes home from a long and traumatic trip. We want them to snap back into domestic life, yet to them a case of chickenpox or a broken dishwasher seems so trivial after witnessing starving children or victims of landmines, say." To this may be added another wife's cache of pent-up irritations. "They fill the house with loads of stinking kit. Sometimes they even give you infectious, unpleasant tropical diseases. They dominate all social occasions with endless retelling of adventures at the front. Lots of voyeuristic descriptions of violence in inappropriate situations."

Mistakes are frequently made by both journalists and partners in a constant cycle of resented separation and fraught reunion. "It took a real, concerted effort to understand how to readjust to life back home," one photographer explained. "It was foolish to bring the war back. It was stupid to expect people here to empathize with you; to even make the attempt was more frustrating than anything else. Not that I wouldn't tell my girlfriend what happened. But only people exposed to that event, and it is a location-specialized thing, could grasp the essence of it. And I think she just thought it was better not to talk to me about life at home because I wouldn't be able to relate to it. I realize now that I should have made more of an effort to talk to her about this. When you actually returned home, the decompression thing was always a problem because I would just need time to readjust on my own. I did not know how to do it properly with somebody else. So I just alienated my partner."

Another recurring theme expressed by the stay-at-home partners was, understandably, safety. To offset her own anxiety, one wife reached an unusual arrangement with her journalist husband. "Before we got married," she explained, "we decided that if my husband did conflict coverage, we would go together. So far, he's been pretty good about it. However, even when he does local assignments I am a nervous wreck and often imagine the worst."

Another wife raised concerns around the safety of a family accompanying a journalist posted on long-term assignment to a dangerous region. "I feel that it is often very stressful for the partners of foreign journalists to live in an alien environment. We lived in Africa for four years. My husband was usually away, and as a family we were often scared not just for my husband but of the constant threat of violence at home. One wife always slept with her children as she was too scared to let them sleep alone."

A further cause for spousal worry is the mental state of some of the journalists on their return from the front lines. War journalists may bring back not just the detritus of war but also the troubling behavioral manifestations of PTSD, depression and heavy drinking. Having spent weeks fretting about the physical safety of their husbands, wives may end up doing little more than exchanging one set of concerns for another. And all the while, there are bills to pay, the heating to fix, a car to service, homework to supervise, birthday parties to organize, sleepless nights tending children with fevers, a career to manage, if it hasn't been placed on hold, and anxious in-laws to placate. The domestic situation becomes particularly unsettled when the war journalist lacks the necessary insight not only into his own state of mind but also into the inordinate pressures faced by his partner. Because such spouses are faced with a plethora of challenges in their relationships, it did not come as a surprise when I received this gratuitous piece of advice from a disheartened wife: "Don't ever be tempted to marry one!"

Some partners of journalists live with the anticipation of tragedy, yet when death arrives it does so unexpectedly. Others simply block their minds to the profession's many dangers. "When my husband went away to cover war zones, I had great (misconceived as it turned out) confidence that he would keep his head down—in effect, I would deny the fact he was in danger," one wife wrote. "He in turn would blithely reassure me by claiming cowardice." Three women who took part in my study had had partners who were murdered. Their deaths were no accident of war, the result of a stray bullet, a missile off target, a bomb gone awry. Each had been deliberately targeted and killed. I did not have an opportunity to interview these women. My understanding of their situation is based therefore on the results from their questionnaires plus their written comments sent to me. What they went through exceeded bereavement. All became depressed and suicidal, and two required antidepressant medication. One woman revealed, "My grief was (and still is, five years later) compounded by the fact that at the time I was pregnant with our daughter. Caring for a small person meant so much of my own feelings had to be put on hold—in itself a 'coping' strategy, as I made her my absolute priority and she in turn became my lifeline."

"No story is worth dying for." I heard this statement repeatedly from those in the news business, and yet journalists continue to die, leaving behind their partners and children and children yet to be born. Their youth, the violent manner of their dying, the talent lost, the arbitrariness of the event, the difficulty in bringing the killers to justice, the logistics of dealing with death in a foreign, hostile land all complicate the bereavement process, bequeathing a residue of intense sadness.

———

My data did reveal one protective factor in a relationship. Journalists often marry journalists. This phenomenon, called assortative mating, is not unique to the profession, and chance cannot account for it. When birds of a feather flock together, there is often a biochemical underpinning to this mutual attraction. Zuckerman's theories of sensation-seeking behavior driven by dopamine and MAO provide the clue. Indeed, there is empirical evidence to show that should partners be incompatible when it comes to searching out new experiences, their relationship may founder. In my data, over a quarter of the war journalists had married another journalist, and it was in this group that the least psychological distress was found.

This chapter has focused on women as war journalists, domestic journalists, wives, partners and widows. However, it is important not to lose sight of the fact that from a behavioral perspective, female war journalists stand apart. Their predilection for living intensely, and often dangerously, is unique to this group. From the enclaves of Bosnia to the jungles of the Congo, from the back alleys of Gaza to the disfigured landscape of Sierra Leone, they have matched their male counterparts in confronting the perils of war to get an important story or telling picture. Indeed, Thomas de Waal, in his introduction to Anna Politkovskaya's book on the Chechen struggle, *A Dirty War*, notes that many of the best journalists in that most dangerous of conflicts have been women, and he mentions specifically Carlotta Gall, Petra Prochazkova, Yelena Masyuk, Maria Eismont and the late Nadezhda Chaikova (murdered in Chechnya in 1996). Female journalists working in zones of conflict may be fewer in number, but the type of work they do and their psychological fortitude in the face of great adversity dispels any notion that they are interlopers in a male domain.

Single, articulate, mentally resilient, an inner physical toughness, competitive, insouciant, can drink with the boys—as applicable as all these descriptors are, they fail to convey the overarching impression created by these women. That defining essence is instead best summed up by the reaction of Marie Colvin to her close brush with death while reporting on the Tamil Tigers in Sri Lanka. "I am not going to hang up my flak jacket as a result of this incident," she wrote in the *Sunday Times*. "I have been flown to New York, where doctors are going to operate on my injured eye. They have told me it is unlikely I will regain much use of it as a piece of shrapnel went right through the middle. All I can hope for is a bit of peripheral vision. Friends have been phoning to point out how many famous people are blind in one eye. They seem to do fine with only one eye, so I am not worried. But what I want most as soon as I get out of hospital is a vodka martini and a cigarette."

7

DOMESTIC JOURNALISTS AND URBAN TERROR: THE AFTERMATH OF SEPTEMBER 11

Men never do evil so completely and cheerfully as when they do it from religious conviction.

— BLAISE PASCAL

On a bright autumnal September morning I was doing a ward round on a psychiatry unit. Situated in a crumbling wing of an old veterans' hospital, the ward, like many psychiatric facilities dating from the Second World War era, has a rundown, decrepit feel to it. A sparsely furnished room, with stained and ripped upholstery and drapes that hang limp and shut unevenly, serves as a patient lounge with messages and poems penned on the walls, and in one corner sits that ever-present appliance that seldom rests, the television set.

To those who have no interest in the observation and study of mental phenomena, the ward may seem a sad place, a way station for the forlorn and forgotten of society. Prey to their delusions, hallucinations and manias, many of these patients have ceded reality to a cornucopia of fantastical beliefs that preoccupy thoughts, affect emotions and dictate actions. How can it be otherwise, when you are convinced that your food has been poisoned by your neighbors, or you believe that the police have inserted a microchip into the recesses of your brain to control what you say, or you hold a grievance against the authorities for incarcerating you with a bunch of madmen simply because you have evidence, incontrovertible proof in fact, that you are nothing less than the Messiah and all you have to do to prove it is to fast for forty days and forty nights, instead of which the bastards send around a van with a bunch of goons, and the next thing you know you wake up in this shithole where doctors, or they call themselves that anyway, ask you absurd questions like, do you ever hear voices?

Overwhelmed by psychosis, these people care not one iota that inflation is up, Milosevic awaits trial in The Hague, Lance Armstrong has won a fourth consecutive Tour de France. Nor does it matter that there is no money in the bank, no housing to be had, no family members who visit. Simply arrest the neighbor, get the surgeon to remove the implanted brain chip, and all will be resolved. Anything less is of no consequence. People mill around in the lounge, oblivious to each other's private torment. Another routine day in state-sponsored purgatory is how one of my patients described his existence here.

On that sunlit September morning the television was on, as usual, although the volume was muted. I was chatting to a patient, listening to his tale of how the physicist Edward Teller had stolen his ideas and claimed credit for developing the H-bomb. Out of the corner of my eye I saw a plane drift lazily across the TV screen and sink into one of the twin towers of the World Trade Center. My patient had seen it too. "Crazy pilot," he muttered, before resuming his complaint of dark deception.

A nurse burst into the room. "Have you heard? Have you heard? A plane has crashed into the World Trade Center. It's on the TV, look!" She pointed excitedly at the screen as colleagues joined her, obscuring the view.

Unfazed by the gathering commotion, my patient hardly broke stride. Teller was a fraud, Teller had stolen intellectual property, Teller had ruined his life, Teller was not even a real physicist, he was an impostor, a cunning charlatan who had fooled the world.

I had heard this all before, countless times, but by now my attention had been distracted by events unfolding on the television. I stood to get a better view. Teller's phantom victim stood too, not to follow the breaking story but to continue his harangue. The drama of the moment was lost on him. I noted that the other three psychotic patients in the room were oblivious to events too. Two sat slumped in chairs, looking vacuous, while a third shuffled around aimlessly, picking up a magazine and skimming desultorily through it. By now the TV's sound had been switched on, with volume on high, making conversation difficult. Undeterred, my patient continued his monologue: a conspiracy among Hungarians, East European nepotism with Teller as the arch puppeteer. He made this last point just before news came through that the Pentagon had been hit.

The room was filling rapidly with nurses, secretaries, physicians all jostling for space in front of the box. I moved off toward a window, between two chairs occupied by patients lost in thought. A corridor of space there presented an acutely angled view of the screen. Smoke and flames were all I could see. Undeterred, my patient shadowed me, his back to the television, and once more my view was obscured. In 1956 Hungarian secret files were taken by the Russians when their tanks rolled into Budapest. That's where Teller gave his game away, where he revealed his true colors, his loyalty to himself only, and in the confusion of the uprising, Teller, devious, loathsome Teller switched documents and assumed my patient's identity, and for forty-four years this man had lived with the doppelgänger who had stolen his life, his brain, his ideas, his family, swindled him out of his inheritance and as a final indignity driven him into the asylum where he continued the persecution by controlling the physicians, paying them on the quiet, oh yes, on the quiet to keep him locked away where no one would believe him. Just because Teller was not a physicist did not make him any less clever. He was unbelievably clever, devious, cunning, scheming, able to switch identities, in fact: he fooled the Russians, the Americans, the Canadians. He was so fucking clever he could turn goulash into hamburgers if he wanted to and the only person who had ever seen through him was ...

I knew what was coming but never did hear it. The collective gasps and shouts from the staff in front of the screen drowned out my patient's *idée fixe*. The second tower had been hit. I had heard enough of Edward Teller and needed to see what was going on. Maneuvering my way into position I stared disbelievingly at the screen in a room that had become eerily silent save for the broadcaster's commentary. We stood awhile transfixed, our work at a standstill as we watched the second tower collapse. Belief suspended, we watched the first tower come down soon after. Little was said. We were all too stunned.

It becomes hard to gauge the passage of time when so engrossed. Perhaps twenty minutes had passed—I cannot be certain—when I became aware that the Teller tirade had abated. To my surprise I noticed my patient too was riveted by events unfolding on the screen. And a second man, whose schizophrenia had long rendered him aloof and disdainful of everything but his monomania, had roused himself from his stupor to follow events. Swept up in the agony of the moment and for that briefest window in time, staff and patients were united in their collective incredulity. In an environment where the reality of physicians clashed daily with the delusions of their patients, it had taken a cataclysm to bring about this tenuous unanimity.

Those horrific images of September 11 did something that neither my verbal interventions nor medication had, up until then, achieved. It had distracted one psychotic patient from an all-embracing delusion and roused another from his state of profound indifference and, for this briefest interlude, brought them back into the world of sound judgment, empathy and numbed disbelief. It was, of course, no cure for their schizophrenia, but remarkable nonetheless. An outrage of startling ferocity had momentarily reawakened these patients' blighted humanity, overriding their faulty neurotransmitters, dysfunctional receptors and altered cerebral blood flow that lay at the root of their psychoses. It remains for me a powerful, enduring memory of that fateful, beautifully clear September morn, and the paradox was striking. An act of moral insanity had restored, albeit briefly and in circumscribed fashion, part of my patients' sheltered realities. "Tsk," muttered my patient, finally turning away from the hypnotic images, "you have to be really crazy to do a thing like that."

―――――

In earlier chapters, the emphasis has been on journalists who travel to foreign shores in search of stories and pictures of conflict. Driven by a complex set of motivations, these men and women have stood apart from their colleagues because of their unique demographic profile and higher levels of psychological distress. In contrast, the domestic journalists used as control subjects have led different lives. Although called on to cover emotionally disturbing stories such as murders and traffic accidents, domestic journalists rarely confront situations of grave personal danger. This was reflected in their lower scores for depression and post-traumatic stress disorder. While they are as driven as their war counterparts to cover the news, get the scoop and make deadlines, their desire to enter zones of conflict is conspicuously absent. War holds no attraction. It is something that happens far from their civil society, and it is best left to others of different temperament to tell the public about it.

And then one morning everything changes. Mars makes a home visit. Suddenly, violently, events that have for generations been viewed as foreign, faraway conflagrations in godforsaken places

arrive in the very heart of a great power's most populous and sym-
bolic cities. Journalists who have, by choice, shied away from war
and the accompanying slaughter can avoid it no longer. Skyscrapers
were leveled, thousands killed, the Pentagon was ablaze and soon
killer microbes would be on the loose. Middle East fanaticism
ceased to be a foreign affair and became the all-encompassing
domestic story. For days on end, as the events of September 2001
unfolded, a group of journalists unaccustomed to mass destruction and death witnessed apocalyptic scenes and confronted the
distraught and bereaved.

How would they cope psychologically with this situation? By
nature more cautious and risk averse than their war colleagues,
these journalists had never been tested by traumatic events of such
magnitude. There were early clues that they found the aftermath of
the attacks emotionally overwhelming. The public, accustomed to
viewing journalists as dispassionate bringers of bad news, was
now confronted by the new phenomenon of reporters crying while
broadcasting live. In one highly publicized incident, the veteran
CBS news anchor Dan Rather broke down while on air, prompting
a debate about the importance of a journalist's maintaining his
professional sangfroid no matter how disturbing the content of the
story. Yet if someone with the experience of Rather was reacting
that way, others in the profession were likely to be affected too.

I therefore thought it would be interesting to study the psychological responses of a group of domestic journalists who had to
cover the events of September 11. The management of CNN was
approached with the suggestion of extending the original journalist study into the domestic domain. They were sympathetic to the
request, and a list of sixty-four names of CNN journalists from
the New York, Washington and Atlanta bureaus was forwarded to
me. The methodology remained essentially the same: a Web site
was set up with a series of questions eliciting basic demographic
data, details pertaining to September 11 and the anthrax attacks as
well as inventories for post-traumatic stress disorder and depres-

sion. One difference was that journalists were not interviewed face to face as in the war study, so no diagnosis of the full PTSD or major depression syndromes could be made.

The forty-six journalists who agreed to take part did not differ in age, gender or location—three important variables that could have potentially influenced PTSD scores—from the eighteen who refused. This suggested that the 72 percent who said yes to the study were truly representative of all the staff involved in covering the terrorist attacks. To provide a way of interpreting the behavioral responses, two sets of control subjects were chosen from previously collected data. The first was a group of forty-five war journalists and the second forty-five domestic journalists whose responses had been gathered well before September 11. None of the latter group had worked in zones of conflict. Once again, care was taken to ensure that these three groups of journalists (the war group and the two domestic groups) were well matched on four variables that could have influenced their PTSD scores, namely age (the average age was late thirties), sex (60 percent male), marital status (50 percent single), and the numbers of years worked as a journalist (an average of fifteen years).

In comparing the psychological responses of war journalists with those of their domestic colleagues pressed into covering the aftermath of the September 11 attacks, there is a risk in blurring the margins between disparate sets of events. The al-Qaeda attacks were quickly interpreted by President George W. Bush and many of the news organizations as America's "new war." At face value this makes comparisons between journalists of different temperamental bents of interest. But the researcher must avoid getting swept up in the emotion of rhetoric. To the behavioral scientist, objectivity is paramount. Without this essential requirement, the interpretation of data, indeed the very collection of the data, becomes tainted and any conclusions may smack of propaganda. War is a small word with a multiplicity of big meanings. It is not necessary here to open a debate over semantics or whether a terrorist attack on the

American mainland equates with the more conventional conflicts the United States has become involved in. What is required
is an attempt to differentiate between the level of danger, the degree
of threat faced by domestic journalists thrust involuntarily and
briefly into conflict and war journalists who, by choice, have
reported on foreign conflict over a period of a decade or more.

To this end, it is helpful to recall the list of stressors confronted
by the group of domestic journalists during the latter third of 2001.
September 11 saw the coordinated air attacks on New York and
Washington, with another hijacked plane crashing into the Penn-
sylvania countryside after passengers stormed the cockpit. In the
months that followed, anthrax became the new terror, with news
organizations one of the selected targets of whoever was distribut-
ing the powder. The offices of NBC in New York had to be vacated
while men in space-age protective clothing probed the environment for the dreaded spores. And then in November, an American
Airlines plane crashed in Queens, with hundreds more killed.

Throughout, the media fulfilled an essential public service,
keeping the citizens informed. To do so demanded regular exposure to scenes of grief, fear, uncertainty, anger and helplessness. To
a degree, these were offset by the resilience and fortitude of survivors and rescue workers, but the overwhelming emotions associated with the attacks by planes and anthrax were pain and sorrow.
The intensity of experiences, the sheer volume of news generated,
the constantly evolving homeland security concerns in the United
States and the unique nature of the biological agents targeting their
profession produced a constellation of stressors unusual in the
history of North American journalism. And for the most part it fell
to the domestic correspondent, photographer, broadcaster and
cameraman to weather the threats, collate the facts and sift through
the fraught and jumbled emotions of the moment, all the while
managing their own fears and feelings.

The targets chosen by the terrorists on September 11, 2001, were symbols of American financial and military power. Shocking as the events were, civil society in the United States did not implode along with the twin towers. Just the contrary—the institutions of state mobilized positively and quickly to deal with trauma's aftermath. The world's richest nation activated a network of support services of mind-boggling proportions—or so it must have seemed to those in less fortunate, long-suffering nations crushed by war and years of strife. The domestic journalists called on to cover events of September 11 may have done so amid the detritus of shattered buildings and shattered lives, but they were also surrounded by functioning cities, water in the taps, sewage taken care of, food aplenty in a bewildering array of restaurants, the lights of Fifth Avenue undimmed and foundations and corporations pouring in millions of dollars in relief aid to supplement the billions promised by the president.

Contrast this with the description of life in a Balkan city by the *New York Times* journalist Chris Hedges. "Sarajevo in the summer of 1995 came close to Dante's inner circle of hell," he wrote. "The city, surrounded by Serb gunners on the heights above, was subjected to hundreds of shells a day, crashing into an area twice the size of Central Park. Multiple Katyusha rockets—whooshing overhead—burst in rapid succession; they could take down a four or five story apartment building in seconds, killing or wounding everyone inside. There was no running water or electricity and little to eat; most people were subsisting on a bowl of soup a day. It was possible to enter the besieged city only by driving down a dirt track on Mount Igman, one stretch directly in the line of Serb fire. The vehicles that had failed to make it lay twisted and upended in the ravine below, at times with the charred remains of their human cargo inside. Families lived huddled in basements, and mothers, who had to make a mad dash to the common water taps set up by the United Nations, faced an excruciating choice—whether to run through the streets with their children or leave them in a building that might be

rubble when they returned. The hurtling bits of iron fragmenta-
tion from exploding shells left bodies mangled, dismembered,
decapitated. The other reporters and I slipped and slid in their
blood and entrails thrown out by the shell blasts, heard the groans
of anguish, and were for our pains in the sights of the Serb snipers,
often just a few hundred yards away. The latest victims lay with
gaping wounds untended in the corridors of hospitals that lacked
antibiotics and painkillers. By that summer, after nearly four years
of fighting, forty-five foreign reporters had been killed, scores
wounded. I lived—sheltered in a side room in the Holiday Inn—its
front smashed and battered by shellfire—in a world bent on self-
destruction, a world where lives were snuffed out at random."

What befell New York and Sarajevo deserves closer comparison
if one is to make sense of the data collected from journalists reporting each city's travails. Both occupied an elevated niche within their
respective societies, Manhattan as the flagship of capitalism's tri-
umphant ascendancy, cosmopolitan Sarajevo as a unique blend of
urbanized Balkan chic and multicultural harmony that had hosted
a recent winter Olympics. These superficial similarities extended
to the violence visited on them: many killed, buildings leveled,
thousands bereaved and traumatized. But the manner in which
this came about differed considerably between sites. The attacks
on New York were unexpected, sudden, the damage inflicted
within a brief period, a morning's mayhem. Death came quickly to
thousands and the wounded were few. The physical damage was
circumscribed—apart from the devastation at the site of the World
Trade Center, the remainder of the city was unscathed physically.
Sarajevo, on the other hand, was ravaged, slowly, piecemeal over
the course of years, a steady, deadly attrition that claimed a daily
quota of casualties, insidiously destroying families, homes, schools,
hospitals, health care, sanitation, the very infrastructure that had
elevated the city to Olympian heights. This unrelenting destruction, on any one day less in magnitude than that inflicted on New
York on September 11, continued unabated over many years. The

cumulative effect on the city and its inhabitants was ruinous. By the time the Dayton accords brought an uneasy, mistrustful peace, a bereaved populace was left to survey their blighted conurbation and wonder where and how to find the will to rebuild their splintered lives.

Sarajevo can stand symbolically for countless other besieged cities. The end point of any protracted warfare is predictably uniform: full cemeteries, empty stores, apathetic, dependent survivors adrift among the remnants of civil society. Chechnya, Rwanda, the Congo, Sierra Leone, Lebanon, Afghanistan, Iraq may all be substituted for the Balkans, the fate of their cities analogous to that of Sarajevo. Horrific as the events of September 11 were, terrible as the fate was of those trapped in the twin towers, by the time the dust settled on that surreal day, New York away from the circumscribed, encapsulated rubble of Ground Zero bore little resemblance to those cities. Which meant that the domestic journalists who were pressed, by circumstance and necessity, into gathering the news from New York confronted a terrain both superficially similar to and fundamentally different from that faced by Hedges and his colleagues as they navigated the lottery of snipers' alley in Sarajevo. The forty-five dead foreign journalists in the Balkans underscore this gulf. These similarities and differences in personal experiences, linked as they inextricably are to the environment in which the journalists function, will help explain the domestic journalists' psychological responses to covering the events of September 11.

———

Of the forty-six journalists in my study, nineteen had covered the breaking story from Ground Zero, seventeen had been in the newsroom and ten were roving reporters, gathering news from many different sources. Two journalists had been wounded in the attack, while one-third of the group studied knew someone who had been killed or injured. In early January 2002, I visited the New York bureau of CNN to meet with a dozen of the study participants. A few were carrying overt emotional scars. It was soon apparent that everyone knew who these individuals were and deferred to them when discussing and interpreting events. Those journalists who had had psychological difficulties in the immediate aftermath of the attacks were surprisingly naive about the origin of their distress. In this, their responses were reminiscent of those of some war journalists. The sudden sprouting of an intense dysphoria coupled with fear bordering on paranoia was misinterpreted as a sign of incipient insanity.

"At CNN we have a deck outside on the twenty-second floor that looks right at downtown," one journalist told me. "I was downtown and witnessed the buildings falling. And then I heard planes overhead and panicked at first, thinking we were going to be attacked as well. I was feeling very vulnerable and so was relieved to see the planes were our military. That evening I would not go home. I was not going to go into Penn Station on a train in a tunnel. I was afraid we would be trapped. I was happy my office put me up in a hotel so I could delay going through the tunnel. Even now, I still have difficulties going through tunnels or crossing a bridge."

The role of many domestic journalists had undergone a profound change. The job expectations were still there, albeit more intense and under pressure. "My office put me up in a hotel for four hours to get some sleep later that night (midnight to 4 a.m.)," recalled an editor. "And then I was back at work for two straight days, looking at video over and over." But now some of the journalists, because of their proximity to Ground Zero and the Armory, assumed the role of comforter to the thousands of relatives and friends searching for missing loved ones. Some journalists were caught in the spotlight by virtue of a miraculous escape from the crumbling towers, none more so than David Handschuh, of the *Daily News* and president of the National Press Photographers Association, whose leg was shattered by falling masonry. Others found they were the focus of a story because of their inability to control their emotions while on the air. "They Can Cry If They Want To. Chris Cramer, CNN President, Salutes the Tearful Urban War Correspondent" ran a headline in a London broadsheet, the *Independent*. And then there were the journalists who simply put their humanity first. This was their city that had been scarred, their neighbors who wandered the streets in numbed bewilderment clutching photographs. They knew the children of parents whose cars had been left standing long after the last commuter train had run.

Miriam Falco, senior producer for CNN medical news, gave compassionate voice to the new roles that many journalists were called on to adopt. "I produced live shots and packages from outside the Armory in New York, where families and friends gathered to find out if their loved ones were alive and later to drop off DNA evidence for identification purposes. We met with a lot of people who were in shock or beginning the grieving process and yet still hoping that their loved ones somehow miraculously survived. Was I on the front lines of the war? No. Was I at Ground Zero, where the destruction and demise of thousands of people were blatantly obvious? No. But I saw the thousands of people pouring past our liveshot location, searching for their loved one, sharing their pictures and stories about those missing, hoping when there was really no way anyone could have survived. It may not sound like a difficult assignment, but it certainly was not easy hearing the accounts of those devastated people. What helped me and my correspondent get through this was knowing that simply listening to their stories, even if they never made the air, provided a little bit of comfort and catharsis for the individual sharing memories of a missing/lost relative or friend. Another factor, which was reflected in our reporting but also provided some 'therapeutic' balance for me, was seeing the countless kind gestures from strangers who flocked to the Armory and anonymously dropped off aid, handing out flowers to the grieving, passing out Hugs candies to anyone passing by, cab drivers refusing to take payment, and so on."

To some journalists, the catastrophe that befell their fellow New Yorkers was disturbingly reminiscent of foreign events they had made a conscious decision to avoid. "I had previously been in war-reporting situations in Central America in the early 1980s and in Afghanistan under the Soviet occupation in the late 1980s," a domestic journalist wrote to me. "The Afghan experience was one that in particular had left me with some post-traumatic stress difficulties. In fact, seeing people die and being under fire led me to stop wanting to chase wars as part of my occupation. Seeing too much of man's inhumanity is corrosive to the human spirit." For this journalist the rapidity and destructive force of the events of September 11 conjured up memories of another kind of trauma. "I would say that the 9/11 events were different in a number of ways: the unexpected, shock nature of it. And also the impact it had on a wide variety of people that I knew. It reminded me more of the Kobe earthquake in Japan that I covered, an event that reverberated for months after." And yet even here the analogy fails. Equating a natural disaster with the events of September 11 misses the essence of what made the attacks on the World Trade Center and the Pentagon so troubling. Unlike the Kobe earthquake, or those in Armenia and Mexico City that preceded it, what occurred on September 11 was no natural disaster, no "act of God," despite the crowing of those fundamentalists who saw it as such. Coupled with grief came the knowledge that the cataclysm was a carefully conceived and daring manifestation of unbridled and, to a naive populace, barely credible, hatred. In life violently taken, there is no victim hierarchy. The dead are pitied equally, accorded the same degree of respect. It is, however, in the manner of the dying that a horror differential is established. Shock and revulsion lie along a sliding scale and crescendo according to the deed. Car crash, train crash, jetliner crash, Lockerbie, Srebrenica, Kigali, reaching an apogee with Auschwitz and the Holocaust. The events of September 11 belong in the upper echelons of a cabal of terror and it fell to domestic journalists immersed in those events to tell the story as it unfolded.

"One of our journalists was downtown at the time of the World Trade Center attacks and saw people jumping out of windows," another producer recalled. "We let her take some time off immediately, but she has had some lingering emotional trouble. And since then there have been a couple of occasions when events such as the accidental plane crash in Queens have had a number of staffers upset and very emotional. Some of our staff folk whom I would put in the 'hardened New Yorker' category from time to time have tears well up, often while watching stories of victims' families and sometimes even while seeing stories not related to the attacks. I am not sure where this fits into the whole analysis of things, but it is real and it's continuing. Everybody puts on a brave face. This is CNN, after all, and the news *does* continue, but folks are more brittle overall now. And it does take a lot of my time to try to figure out ways to smooth things out for my staff."

Informative as it was to hear from individual journalists, I had no way of gauging whether those present in the room were representative of the bureau as a whole. I would have to wait for the group data before any trends became apparent. Over a period of four to five months following September 11, the data were collected.

The PTSD results provided unequivocal, empirical evidence that from a psychological perspective, domestic journalists were adversely affected by the terrorist atrocities. This was most obvious in New York–based journalists, but it was not limited to them. Domestic journalists of all types post–September 11 had significantly more PTSD symptoms than domestic journalists pre–September 11. Now their PTSD profile resembled more closely that of the war journalists. Indeed, with respect to the PTSD triad the scores of the two groups overlapped. When the analysis was extended beyond the three subscales to the twenty-two individual symptoms of PTSD, only one statistically significant difference was found—the domestic journalists had higher hypervigilance scores than those in the war group.*

To better understand these findings, we need to revisit some of the theory underpinning PTSD. In response to a sudden and overwhelming traumatic event a person may develop a hitherto-dormant sense of heightened personal vulnerability. The traumatic event shatters a cocoon of inviolability that has never been questioned, and in response newfound fears and uncertainties quickly take hold. If the unthinkable could happen once, people tell themselves, what is to stop it from happening again? This question holds a compelling logic. Having been exposed and therefore sensitized to violence, the body's nervous system readjusts to the threat recently posed. In this state of increased arousal, pulse and respiratory rates quicken, blood pressure rises and the senses become more acute. Sleep, a period of vulnerability when physical and emotional defenses are down, is affected. Typically, recently traumatized persons describe difficulty falling asleep simply because their "early warning system" refuses to switch off, which would be to let the guard down. Insomnia ensues. But the body cannot maintain this state indefinitely, for sustained amplified awareness is associated with an outpouring of hormones like cortisol, which are helpful in the short term but injurious thereafter. In response to this altered physiology, difficulties with concentration become apparent, and the combination of sleep-deprived nights and stress-filled waking hours produces irritability and outbursts of anger.

Nothing validates the expectation of further dangers more than a new, very real threat. In the wake of the collapse of the twin towers, these were not long in coming, and many targeted the media. "Two

---

* The question posed was, Do you feel watchful and on guard? In the aftermath of the September 11 attacks, more domestic journalists said yes.

days after the attack, we had a bomb threat clear our building," one participant told me. "Some journalists refused to return to the office for a week after that." This was followed by anthrax-laced mail arriving in the post. The threat had shifted from incendiary jetliners to microspores, invisible, silent, odorless but no less lethal. A constant wariness of fresh dangers exemplifies the responses of journalists covering the September 11 attacks and their aftermath.

While the above explanation accords well with trauma theory and makes intuitive sense, the reasons for the increased PTSD scores among the domestic journalists defied such neat categorization. Difficulties with sleep and concentration, irritability and newfound strains in relationships, while all part of PTSD, are not unique to the disorder. Other factors—epiphenomena of the attacks—were also affecting how the journalists responded to the questionnaires. Considerable stress was generated simply by the sheer volume of news. "Immediately after the attacks, the demands for more work were very heavy," one respondent told me. "Near round-the-clock coverage from New York meant a lot of our staffers were pressed into service on other programs." Another journalist said, "Like many of my colleagues, I actually enjoy the challenge of reporting/producing under pressure. This is a huge story. It's why we became journalists in the first place. I would say that most of my current stresses (less sleep, a bit more edgy) are due to the intense focus and long hours on a single story. I have cut back on outside activities, let bills pile up and with the exception of two weekends away have spent virtually all my waking hours in the past few months focused on *the* story. But, I am aware I need a break."

Ironically, the very traits of dogged persistence and perpetual curiosity that make successful journalists may have unforeseen drawbacks. The public's hunger for news, the competition among news agencies for a dramatic story, the individual quest for a scoop, the endless replaying of video footage before deciding what to air all combine to hold journalists captive to events that may be painful to witness or listen to. The thermostat of emotional comfort is set individually, not collectively. Like their war colleagues, the domestic journalists each respond differently to traumatic and stressful events. Apply enough pressures, and symptoms of psychological distress become increasingly frequent. And in some cases, unexplained medical symptoms arise, as with the war journalist with the pseudo stroke or the stammering speech of the young Ugandan girl whose freelance journalist father had been shot. Following September 11, domestic journalists found themselves susceptible to similar conversion symptoms. A letter from one of the participants in my study described his physical difficulties: "About five days after the attacks, my hours were changed to help out on other shows. A few days later I developed a horrible pain in my left shoulder. I am left-handed and had just finished training hard for a triathlon. In light of the attacks, the triathlon was canceled. Anyway, my point is this: I was at peak fitness and was ready for the competition but developed this ailment. I could not turn a doorknob or hold a pen, it was so painful. I tried to make a doctor's appointment, but the earliest I could be seen was in two weeks. Within three days, the pain went away on its own. It is possible it was from overstraining, but I feel stress was the reason for the pain." In a similar vein, a second journalist wrote, "I've accepted the probability that my recent physical ailment could be the direct result of the events of September 11." The displacement of psychological distress into physical symptoms, the conversion of unconscious feelings and emotions into weakness, pain and immobility, was not reported by a single domestic journalist among the 107 studied well before September 11.

Interestingly, domestic journalists post–September 11 were not significantly depressed; their scores on the twenty-one-item Beck Depression Inventory were indistinguishable from their pre-9/11 colleagues and well below those of the war journalists. Here, the New York–Sarajevo comparisons are particularly germane in trying to understand why this should be. For journalists covering the news in New York the threats and dangers were largely ephemeral.

Apart from the anthrax scare, which was quickly contained and for which curative treatment was available, the insecurity was linked to an anticipation of future attacks that never materialized. To be sure, this generated prominent hypervigilance, as my data revealed, but contrast the phantom fears, whipped up in part by the Department of Homeland Security's kaleidoscopic warnings, with the situation in Sarajevo, where anxieties received a daily validation— fresh attacks, new casualties, colleagues wounded and killed. For some war journalists, the effects of relentless siege on mood were corrosive. These stark differences in personal safety were a product of fundamentally different environments, the one with civil society intact, rallying, supportive, restorative, the other with little but the remnants of such a society undefiled, the vestiges in daily peril, disintegrating into a racist abyss familiar to Europeans of an older generation. For some war journalists, the weeks, months and years spent in this resurgent barbarity wasted the spirit, inducing a melancholy in tune with the ravaged surroundings and disconsolate populace.

———

It is of course possible that the signs and symptoms of psychological distress in domestic journalists post–September 11 were simply part of a collective societal angst that gripped many of those living in the greater New York area. A study conducted by New York's Board of Education looked at the cumulative effects of September 11 and the anthrax attacks on children in Grades 4 through 12. It found that approximately 75,000 suffered PTSD, while over 100,000 had developed agoraphobia, a fear of open spaces. In March 2002, an article in the *New England Journal of Medicine* described the prevalence of PTSD among the residents of Manhattan living south of 110th street. Of more than 1,000 adults interviewed, 7.5 percent reported symptoms consonant with the diagnosis, significantly higher levels than those found in the general population.

Furthermore, the authors noted that the rate of PTSD trebled in those residents living south of Canal Street, the area close to the World Trade Center. This link between physical proximity to the attack and the development of PTSD symptoms was mirrored in the data, in that those journalists working in New York had significantly higher PTSD scores than those reporting from elsewhere.

While location was a powerful predictor of whether a person developed PTSD symptoms, the psychological fallout of the al-Qaeda terror was not limited to journalists in the United States. Unforgettable images of jetliners plowing into skyscrapers, people leaping from the upper stories and the ghost-like survivors shrouded in dust staggering from the scene appeared repetitively on television screens around the world. In deciding which pictures to run, staffers in international newsrooms sifted through untold variations on a theme of death. In the process, PTSD-like reactions by proxy were induced in journalists many thousands of miles removed from the scene. One European journalist described to me a plethora of stresses, emotional and physical, that followed in September 11's murky wash. The fact that the journalist had no direct exposure to the trauma does not invalidate her distress, which stemmed in large measure from the concentration of visually disturbing images to which she was subjected. News bosses, in their hubris, should take note. Emollient assurances that all is well with journalists away from the front lines, cloistered in the hothouse shelter of a production room, may prove misleading. Repetitive exposure to dehumanizing acts can exert its own insidious effect on the psyche.

"For the past couple of years I have managed a team that monitors and logs all incoming TV footage," she told me. "We are often confronted with horrendous scenes, which haven't really had much impact on me. Apart from one occasion when I had nightmares, about seven years ago, my attitude has always been that this is part of life, and I have developed a very warped sense of humor to deal with some of the things I have seen. However, the workload has had some negative effects on my physical health.

"On September 11, I worked through till two-thirty the following morning and was back in the office by eight. I continued to work in similar fashion for the next two weeks and was totally exhausted. We were subject to nonstop pictures from a variety of angles and sources. There was no time to eat properly, take a break, see my friends or family, cry, talk it through, pray—all the usual things you do to get it out of your system. For weeks afterward I suffered flashbacks and nightmares about people jumping out of the towers. The image seemed imprinted on my mind. I wasn't sleeping well, and I just couldn't stop working for fear I'd never be able to start again. Finally I came down with some sort of flu bug and had to stop. However, I didn't seem able to kick it, and when I did try to go back to work, I started having panic attacks, going hot and cold and crying at the least thing. At this point my doctor told me I had to rest, gave me some medication and signed me off work for three weeks. Even then I was working from home by logging in, dealing with calls on my mobile and so on.

"It was only when one of my senior managers phoned me full of concern and told me I had to stop and get some rest that I started to calm down. The hardest thing was not watching or listening to any news bulletins and trying to switch off. Eventually I went abroad for a couple of weeks to try to chill out, and I am now back at work. The nightmares and flashbacks have stopped and I'm down to the odd panic attack every few days. Although I am feeling a lot better now I'm still not 100 percent, and it does cross my mind that I will never be able to function properly in my current job. My tolerance level is very low, and I'm even finding social situations hard going. Noise drives me crazy—for example, phones ringing, TV monitors on, general chat.

"I know I will get better. I'm absolutely determined. I realized what was wrong with me as soon as the panic attacks started—and hopefully I'm doing the right things to get better. I do not want the rest of my life to be affected by this—especially the inability to control my body's reactions. I have several friends who have really lost the plot after a number of years working in war zones with several near misses, and they are a bag of nerves. I do wonder whether if I'd actually been sent out to cover the story I'd be okay—mainly because I'd feel I was helping in some way rather than just having to observe."

———

Three months after the events of September 11, on a chilly winter's evening, I met a Serbian journalist for a drink at a favorite watering hole in Toronto. Having left her homeland during the repressive years of the Milosevic regime, she now resides in England and had come to spend a sabbatical at the Munk Centre for International Studies at the University of Toronto. We perched on our bar stools. The pub was crowded. The wooden paneling, subdued lighting and pints of Guinness invited conversation, and with a predictable inevitability, the topic turned to war and the dismantling of civil society in the Balkans. At first, there was nothing unusual about what we discussed, how ethnic hatred had blighted the region, leaving a legacy of anger, mistrust and above all grief. For the most part I listened while she spoke of broad, sweeping themes, widely debated in the media during the many years of civil war. But gradually her thoughts and recollections became more focused, personal, heartfelt. She talked of Balkan journalists, the archetypal tough guys reporting on a tough war, suddenly finding it difficult to control their emotions. Haunted by memories, perplexed by a vulnerability that was somehow shameful, adrift in a society that lionized strength, they felt too guilty to express their distress when those around them, their own communities, had suffered so much more. As she spoke, this petite, courageous, lively woman was crying, silent tears coursing a gentle slalom over the high color of her cheeks. She began to tell the story of a colleague who, in traveling from one ravaged Bosnian hamlet to another, had come to a clearing in the woods where a local militia had set up camp. Initially, there seemed little amiss. It was a typical camp scene: smoke rising from fires, men lazing about, strips of what appeared to be meat being smoked above a flame. And then, to his stupefaction, the journalist realized that the meat was human flesh. Strips of flesh, cut from the bones of men and women, done not as a descent into cannibalism, for there was food enough, but rather as one further despoliation of the dead, mocking, dehumanizing those who had so recently been neighbors.

There is a troubling incongruity in hearing a tale of such depravity while sitting in the *gemütlich* ambiance of the pub, the barman discreetly attentive to the level in your glass, and outside safe, silent streets and the sparkle of festive bunting on trees. After a tale of smoked human flesh, there is nowhere else for conversation to go. What is there to say? How are you to respond? My guest dabbed her eyes and apologized. I said there is nothing to apologize for. She laughed. It's that Balkan temperament, she joked. Can't show signs of weakness. And then she grew serious once more. "You know, what happened in New York recently was terrible," she said, "too terrible for words. My heart goes out to those people, but maybe now, just maybe, others, like the Americans and the Canadians, can understand what we went through, what it is like to have such trauma, such evil in your society." There was no schadenfreude in this statement, only a lingering sense of sadness.

On the first anniversary of the September attacks, I returned to the offices of CNN in New York. The mood was somber, but quite different from that I had encountered eight months earlier. Few journalists sought me out, and those who did displayed little more than residual anxiety, now well controlled. Some lingering doubts and insecurities persisted, of course, occasionally manifesting as heightened concerns for the safety of their children or disturbing nightmares. One journalist, for example, dreamed of standing atop the twin towers, one foot firmly planted on each intact edifice, while below lay the devastated remains of New York City, every other building flattened exactly the way the World Trade Center had been. But for the most part, the domestic journalists were getting on with their lives. How they will continue to fare psychologically rests largely on what the future holds. Further terrorist attacks of the magnitude of September 11 will challenge some who have already been sorely tried. In the end the greatest threat posed by weapons of mass terror, be they anthrax or commandeered jetliners, may not be the immediate loss of life—which can ultimately be contained—but the psychological toll of high levels of stress and the attrition wrought by an abiding sense of vulnerability, living with fear and in the expectation of future calamity.

AFTERWORD

All I know is just what I read in the papers.

— WILL ROGERS

My interview with a defensive Maggie O'Kane started on a difficult note. "I don't necessarily buy your theory that we are all traumatized," she told me. I assured her that was not my view. And indeed the results of the study proved us both correct. After a decade or more confronting situations that are hazardous in the extreme, some journalists do develop psychological problems such as post-traumatic stress disorder and depression. But they are a minority, albeit a substantial one. This should not be surprising, given what front-line journalists do in war. The more remarkable observation, perhaps, is that the majority emerge relatively unscathed. Through a complex interplay of factors that determine motivation, a self-selection process is at work, ensuring that most journalists who choose conflict as their area enjoy what they do, are very good at it and manage to keep the life-threatening hazards from undermining their psychological health. To be sure, residual distressing symptoms such as troubling dreams, flashbacks and startle responses are commonly found, but they by themselves do not constitute evidence of formal psychiatric illness.

There is, however, one clinically relevant statistic I have not given: journalists who over the course of their careers developed a disorder like PTSD or became seriously depressed seldom received treatment. This neglect, at times approaching disdain, was part of a wider macho culture of silence that historically has enveloped the profession when it came to psychological health and other emotionally freighted issues such as divorce, dysfunctional relationships and alcohol abuse. It helps explain not only the failure to provide treatment but also why a study like mine was not done earlier. While the management of news organizations is partly to blame for this, journalists themselves also played a part, through a combination of naiveté, embarrassment and concern that future career prospects would suffer if news of their emotional distress reached their bosses. It is only over the past few years that attitudes have become more enlightened and informed. Research and education are the means to strip away remaining taboos and misconceptions.

Conscious of the sensitivities of the journalists and their managers to questions that probed their psyches, I was at pains throughout my study to emphasize that my aim was not to pathologize a profession. But it has never been more important to ask the type of questions I do of those who choose war as their workplace. I have never encountered a journalist who did not view his or her profession as highly dangerous. And now there is evidence that these hazards are multiplying. The murder of the *Wall Street Journal* reporter Daniel Pearl provides fresh proof of this. While journalists are divided on whether Pearl miscalculated the risks attached to his story, one respected colleague, Scott Anderson, noted in his *New York Times* article that Daniel Pearl was a careful man who looked out for his safety. "What is haunting to the rest of us," wrote Anderson, "is that there appears no cautionary lesson to be derived from his death, nothing we would have done differently." In the past, journalists have been killed for many reasons: an accidental stray bullet or artillery shell; being mistaken for a combatant; deliberately targeted because a warlord wanted some unsavory truths suppressed. But the death of Pearl, as Janine di Giovanni pointed out in her *Times* article, adds a new, chilling dimension to this list: a journalist murdered by fanatics because of his religion.

In a post–September 11 world, seething with religious and ethnic hatred, it is not difficult to anticipate nationality joining religion as a marker of a heightened, newfound risk. A visit to Jerusalem and the embattled news bureaus there provided me with sad and dispiriting evidence of this. Just off the Old Jaffa Road sits a nondescript three-story building, home to many of the major television news organizations. Even before I made it up into the CNN offices I had repeatedly been given well-meaning but nevertheless alarming advice by the journalists I had come to meet: never take a bus ride; if your taxi stops behind a bus, instruct the driver to move, and if he refuses, get out and walk; make sure your taxi avoids the main bus routes and so on. Foreign journalists may be able to avoid the vehicles that have become symbols of danger and mass death, but escaping altogether from omnipresent terror is not possible. The Canadian Broadcasting Corporation's Neil MacDonald told me that when a suicide bomber blew himself up outside a private, secluded school attended by many of the foreign press corps's children, his severed head catapulted into the schoolyard, coming to rest in front of the horrified pupils. Personal safety and that of dependents is, however, only part of the stress confronted daily by journalists in the Hold Land. Many find themselves vilified by Israelis and Palestinians, this hatred a product of fevered emotions that have ensured both sides regard the news organizations as biased. CNN journalists are derided by the Israelis for their perceived insensitivity in covering the aftermath of suicide bombings, but the Arab world takes the opposite view, mockingly referring to the organization as the "Zionist News Network." As for the local Israeli and Palestinian journalists, they have increasingly gone their separate ways, reflecting the deep schisms that divide their two societies. The longevity of the second intifada only adds to the attrition, divisions and distress.

News organizations are no longer insensitive to these concerns. Corporate culture has begun changing, particularly in broadcasting. Hostile-environment training is now considered mandatory for journalists who choose to work in zones of conflict, and lectures on post-traumatic stress disorder are part of this curriculum. Led by the BBC and CNN, the news agencies Reuters and the Associated Press now provide confidential counseling, as do most of the major networks, including the Canadian and Australian Broadcasting Corporations and the prime American networks, ABC, CBS and NBC. Management is deliberately kept out of this process, thereby protecting the journalist's right to privacy. The situation among the newspapers is, however, very different. While they have adopted, with alacrity, safety training related to chemical and biological warfare, their efforts lag well behind those in broadcasting when it comes to the emotional fallout of the hazards confronted. It is fair to conclude that the majority of editors remain disturbingly unenlightened on these issues that go to the very heart of their employees' well-being.

Any innovative developments that promote an increased awareness of psychological issues are to be welcomed, although here too I must add a cautionary note: journalists cannot be forced or coerced into therapy. Indeed, there is evidence suggesting that mass debriefing of people who have experienced traumatic stressors may, in some cases, do more harm than good by infecting the resilient with the angst of the symptomatic. In a profession that is not for the faint-hearted, such facts take on added salience. In turn, these potential pitfalls must be viewed alongside a considerable body of research demonstrating the effectiveness of medication and certain forms of psychotherapy in treating PTSD and depression.

The way forward should ideally combine an awareness of individual psychological vulnerability with accurate and confidential mechanisms for detecting those in distress. The methodology described in my study is one way of doing this. Once identified, journalists should be offered the option of a voluntary treatment plan tailored to their individual needs. Here it is important to reiterate that disorders such as PTSD and depression exert a heavy toll on those affected, with untreated symptoms usually worsening over time. Conversely, the prognosis improves with timely and appropriate interventions. A few discreet questions as part of an annual medical checkup may be all that is needed to bring potential problems to light. A referral for treatment can follow quickly, with all news organizations having a roster of appropriate specialists to call on.

It is imperative for news organizations to look after the health of their journalists, be it physical or emotional. "The reporter is the last bastion of truth," noted the veteran war journalist Jon Swain on the eve of the American-led invasion to topple Saddam Hussein. If that situation is to endure, every effort should be made to ensure that the facts are not distorted by a journalist's depression, anxiety, substance abuse or post-traumatic stress disorder, for all these conditions may act as a biased filter through which a particular event, emotional in itself, is viewed. To the BBC's Mark Brayne, emotions, trauma and good journalism are inseparable, the quality and credibility of any story or image of war directly dependent on the journalist's state of mind. This should not be misconstrued as an appeal for journalism free of passion and anger, emotions that can generate powerful reportage. But when a journalist is overwhelmed by his or her emotions—when subjective distress clouds judgment and alters perceptions—inaccurate, misleading work may be the result. The last bastion becomes corrupted. The public is misinformed. For a journalist, there can be no greater indictment.

"Man should not try to avoid stress any more than he would shun food, love or exercise," wrote the celebrated stress researcher Hans Selye. War journalists would no doubt loudly concur. Their profession provides ample opportunity to confront and master stressful situations. Even as I write this conclusion, the war in Iraq is winding down and fourteen journalists lie dead, with another two missing and presumed dead. These disturbing statistics confirm, if confirmation was ever needed, that war journalism will never be made safe. Risk can be reduced but never removed. The good war journalists understand this, work to mitigate it and, in some cases, may even welcome it. But as they navigate a path through war's many hazards, they would do well to reflect on what else Selye had to say: "Don't be afraid to enjoy the stress of a full life nor so naive as to think you can do without some intelligent thinking and planning."

It is in a similar light and with an eye on journalists' psychological well-being that I hope my book has been read.

The results of the first psychological study of war journalists were published in the *American Journal of Psychiatry* in September 2002. I have reproduced the article here. It provides the reader with data that were not included in this book.

Appendix

A Hazardous Profession:
War, Journalists, and Psychopathology

Anthony Feinstein, Ph.D., M.D.

John Owen, M.A.

Nancy Blair, M.A.

Objective: War journalists often confront situations of extreme danger in their work. Despite this, information on their psychological well-being is lacking.

Method: The authors used self-report questionnaires to assess 140 war journalists, who recorded symptoms of posttraumatic stress disorder (PTSD) (with the Impact of Event Scale—Revised), depression (with the Beck Depression Inventory-II), and psychological distress (with the 28-item General Health Questionnaire). To control for stresses generic to all journalism, the authors used the same instruments to assess 107 journalists who had never covered war. A second phase of the study involved interviews with one in five journalists from both groups, using the Structured Clinical Interview for Axis I DSM-IV Disorders.

Results: The rates of response to the self-report questionnaires were approximately 80% for both groups. There were no demo-graphic differences between groups. Both male and female war journalists had significantly higher weekly alcohol consumption. The war journalists had higher scores on the Impact of Event Scale and the Beck Depression Inventory. Their lifetime prevalence of PTSD was 28.6%, and the rates were 21.4% for major depression and 14.3% for substance abuse. War journalists were not, however, more likely to receive treatment for these disorders.

Conclusions: War journalists have significantly more psychiatric difficulties than journalists who do not report on war. In particular, the lifetime prevalence of PTSD is similar to rates reported for combat veterans, while the rate of major depression exceeds that of the general population. These results, which need replicating, should alert news organizations that significant psychological distress may occur in many war journalists and often goes untreated.

(Am J Psychiatry 2002; 159:1570–1575)

Journalism can be a hazardous profession. During 2001 alone, 100 journalists were killed and many hundreds imprisoned and maltreated (1). While the majority were local journalists, targeted for exposing corruption or expressing political dissent, the names of foreign war correspondents feature prominently among those killed or detained. It should be self-evident that war is dangerous and that those who report on it run the risk of becoming casualties themselves, a point poignantly made by a collection of photographs of the Vietnam war assembled from the work of photographers killed in the conflict (2). What is new, however, is a perception in the profession that the number of war journalists killed may be on the increase (3). The recent ambush and murder in Sierra Leone of two of the most respected war journalists shocked the industry and demonstrated that experience, knowledge, and common sense are not guarantees of survival.

It is therefore notable that despite the risks inherent in reporting war, we could find no research on the psychological health of war reporters. In the absence of empirical data, eloquent anecdotal evidence remains the only source offering clues as to the mental well-being of war journalists. Ranging from Robert Capa's memoir of World War II (4), through Michael Herr's account of Vietnam (5), to Anthony Loyd's self-revelatory telling of the Balkans tragedy (6), war journalists' accounts have spelled out not only the horrors of conflict, but also the journalists' reactions to the considerable dangers they confront in getting news to the public.

The lack of research in this area contrasts with a burgeoning trauma literature on the emotional effects of combat on soldiers (7, 8) and civilians (9, 10). The psychological consequences of being subjected to life-threatening events include posttraumatic stress disorder (PTSD), major depression, substance abuse, and dissociative disorder, four of the most common and disabling conditions. Similar responses have been documented after both manmade (11, 12) and natural (13, 14) disasters. What all these reports have in common is the conclusion that individuals will develop an array of psychopathology in response to situations of great personal danger.

Given the dearth of data in relation to war journalists, coupled with concerns that reporting war may be becoming increasingly dangerous, we investigated the extent and nature of psychopathology among those who bring us the news from the world's conflict zones.

Method

We approached six major news organizations—CNN, BBC, Reuters, CBC, Associated Press, ITN (Independent Television News)—and an organization representing freelance journalists (the Rory Peck Trust) and explained the purposes of the study. All of the organizations agreed to participate and provided 170 names, together with work and e-mail addresses. Only journalists fluent in English and currently covering war were assessed.

First Phase

The first phase of the study involved asking the journalists to complete a series of self-report questionnaires. The itinerant nature of war journalism, the far-flung geographic locations involved, and the fact that postal services frequently stop during periods of conflict made contacting the journalists problematic. To overcome this difficulty, we developed an interactive web site. Each journalist was assigned an individual, confidential identification number that had to be entered to access the web site. The contents of the paper and Internet versions were identical and covered 1) basic demographic data, 2) details of alcohol and illicit drug use, and 3) assessment of PTSD, depression, psychological distress, and personality traits by four self-report questionnaires.

The basic demographic data included the number of years the respondent had worked as a war journalist, the list of wars covered, and past psychiatric history. Attempts at tallying all traumatic events were abandoned given the impracticality of the task. The average duration of time spent in zones of conflict by the war journalists (approximately 15 years) meant that the hazardous events experienced were too numerous to accurately recall. For example, the one war that attracted the greatest number of war journalists was the Bosnian conflict, which lasted many years. Journalists took to living in cities under siege, such as Sarajevo, where their attempts at reporting or filming the news often exposed them daily to life-threatening situations.

A unit of alcohol was defined as a regular-size bottle of beer, a glass of wine, or a shot of spirits. Fourteen units of alcohol per week for men and 9 units for women were considered the upper limits of acceptable weekly intake (15).

The Impact of Event Scale—Revised (16) contains 22 questions that closely follow the DSM-IV criteria for PTSD. Thus, the questionnaire contains three subscales for intrusive (reexperiencing), avoidance, and hyperarousal phenomena. We followed the rating scale instructions by asking subjects to indicate symptoms that occurred during the past 7 days only and were related to traumatic, dangerous, or disturbing life experiences. Given the many wars covered by the group, we did not specify any particular conflict or event but allowed the journalists to chose single, multiple, or no events, as they deemed suitable. We did, however, ask the journalists to specify what events had been most troubling to them. For all the war journalists, the events chosen related to their war exposure.

The Beck Depression Inventory-II (17), which contains 21 mood-related questions, was used to assess depression. It provides a choice of four responses per question and is scored in a Likert fashion (the possible scores are 0, 1, 2, 3).

The 28-item General Health Questionnaire (18) contains four subscales, each with seven questions, describing symptoms of somatic complaints, anxiety, social dysfunction, and depression, respectively. A choice of four responses is provided for each question. The subscale scores are summed to give an overall index of psychological distress. A simple Likert scoring method (possible scores of 0, 1, 2, 3) was used as this is preferred for detecting between-group differences in subscale scores.

Second Phase

The second phase of the study involved direct interviews. The difficulties in contacting the group were magnified when it came to direct interviews, and because of time and cost restraints, it was not possible to interview the entire study group. Therefore, a random sample of 20% of the responding journalists were approached for interview. None refused. The interviews took place in New York, London, Paris, Madrid, Barcelona, and Johannesburg. The 28 journalists were interviewed with the Structured Clinical Interview for Axis I DSM-IV Disorders (SCID) (19), and the prevalences of PTSD, mood disorders, and substance use disorders (lifetime, current, and before war exposure) were ascertained. The interviewer was blind to the results of the self-report questionnaires.

Comparison Group

Irrespective of setting, there are stressors generic to journalism (e.g., deadlines, "scooping" the competition). To control for these in symptom expression, we assessed a comparison group of non-war journalists. A group of 107 domestic journalists who did not report on war were approached to undergo the same assessment procedure used with the war journalists. While some in this group also occasionally reported on distressing events (e.g., plane crashes), care was taken to exclude those who had traveled to report on war. Similarly, a random sample of 19 of these journalists (18%) were selected for interview with the SCID. None refused. The interviews were conducted face-to-face or by telephone.

Statistical Analysis

We compared the two groups by using t tests and chi-square analyses. All two-by-two chi-square analyses were two-sided and Yates corrected. If any one cell in a two-by-two analysis had a count of less than 5, a two-sided Fisher's exact test was used. With respect to between-group t test analyses, the Levene test for equality of variance was applied, and where appropriate, the unequal-variance t values and significance levels were reported. All t tests were two-tailed. To control for multiple comparisons, we applied a Bonferroni correction (0.05/22, setting the significance level at 0.002). Transmitting data from a web site relied on the variable quality of the Internet connection. In a few cases, this resulted in lost data. Since the number of subjects varied slightly between tests, the results are presented with the relevant numbers of subjects.

Consent

Both the paper and Internet versions of the study received ethical approval. After complete description of the study to the subjects, written informed consent was obtained. On the web site, subjects gave consent by clicking on the "I agree" box after reading the descriptive preamble.

Results

Self-Report Questionnaires

One journalist was murdered before the questionnaire reached him, thereby reducing the number of subjects to 169. Of these, 82.8% (N=140) gave their consent. The response rate in the comparison group was similar, i.e., 79.9% (107 of 134). The war group had spent, on average, 15 years reporting on wars; the list of conflicts covered included every major conflagration during this period, i.e., Bosnia, Rwanda, Chechnya, the Gulf war and Middle East, Congo, Sierra Leone, Indonesia, Somalia, Ethiopia, Afghanistan, and others. The two groups of journalists were well

TABLE 1. Demographic Characteristics of War Journalists and Comparison Journalists Reporting on Other Subjects

Characteristic	War Journalists (N=140)		Comparison Journalists (N=107)		Analysis		
	Mean	SD	Mean	SD	t	df	p
Age (years)	39.2	6.3	39.0	8.2	0.2	192.5	0.84
Length of career as a journalist (years)	15.6	6.8	15.5	8.5	0.1	186.2	0.94
	N	%	N	%	Yates-Corrected χ^2 (two-sided)	df	p
Gender					1.9	1	0.18
Male	110	78.6	76	71.0			
Female	30	21.4	31	29.0			
Marital status					9.2	2	0.01
Single	61	43.6	28	26.2			
Married	64	45.7	69	64.5			
Divorced	15	10.7	10	9.3			

matched with respect to age, gender, and years of work as a journalist (Table 1). An analysis of marital status revealed similar proportions of divorced journalists in the two groups but more unmarried journalists in the war group (Table 1). A reanalysis of marital status with divorced journalists excluded did not reveal a significant group difference (χ^2=9.0, df=1, p=0.003) after Bonferroni correction.

When it came to psychiatric comparisons, the war group performed significantly worse on a number of variables (Table 2). The mean weekly alcohol consumption levels, 14.7 units for men and 10.8 units for women, were two and three times those of the nonwar group, respectively. With 14 units of alcohol per week considered the upper limit of acceptable drinking for men (15), 45 war journalists as opposed to 13 nonwar journalists were drinking excessively (χ^2=11.9, df=1, p=0.001). The comparable numbers of women, at a weekly limit of 9 units, were 15 and two, respectively (p=0.0001, Fisher's exact test, two-sided). There were no differences between groups in use of cannabis or hard drugs.

Psychometric comparisons based on the three rating scales are also displayed in Table 2. Regarding symptoms of PTSD, the war journalists endorsed more symptoms of intrusive thoughts and images of trauma events (all war related in the case of war journalists) while displaying greater avoidance and hyperarousal phenomena. The war journalists had significantly higher scores on the Beck Depression Inventory, and this difference was confirmed by the scores on the depression subscale of the General Health Questionnaire (Table 2).

The war journalists were not significantly more likely to have received psychiatric help; 24.6% (34 of 138) had received psychotropic medication, psychotherapy, or a combination of the two treatments, compared with 16.2% (17 of 105) of the comparison journalists (χ^2=2.6, df=1, p=0.11).

Subject Interviews

Every fifth journalist from the war (N=28) and nonwar (N=19) groups was interviewed. For the war group, lifetime, current, and prewar diagnoses of PTSD were made

for eight (28.6%), three (10.7%), and one (3.6%) subject, respectively. For major depression the numbers were six (21.4%), two (7.1%), and one (3.6%), respectively. For substance abuse the numbers were four (14.3%), two (7.1%), and one (3.6%), respectively. No journalist in the comparison group had had PTSD, while one (5.3%) had a lifetime diagnosis of major depression and one (5.3%) a lifetime diagnosis of substance abuse; in both cases the disorders had begun before the individuals began working as journalists.

Discussion

In this study of 140 war journalists, drawn from the world's major news organizations, we found higher rates of psychopathology than in a demographically matched comparison group of 107 nonwar journalists. Specifically, the war journalists drank more heavily and showed higher rates of PTSD and major depression. They were not more likely to receive treatment for these conditions. Before discussing these results in greater detail, we would like to address the composition of the study group.

Experienced war journalists are relatively few in number. The 170 names forwarded by organizations such as the BBC and CNN represent a sizable segment of those who travel to areas of conflict. Our response rate of greater than 80% therefore suggests our subjects are representative of war journalists in general. The fact they have been reporting wars for, on average, 15 years highlights not only their experience but also our success in capturing the central core of bona fide war journalists, as opposed to those who cover a conflict or two before moving on to less hazardous news work. It is also important to note that while war journalists are never openly forced into covering a particular conflict by their news bosses, it is generally recognized that a pattern of refusing dangerous assignments may have adverse career consequences. Thus, when starting out in their career there is a tendency to accept every war story. Only as established war journalists can they be more selective in choosing when and where they are sent.

TABLE 2. Psychiatric Measures for War Journalists and Comparison Journalists Reporting on Other Subjects

Measure	War Journalists (N=140)		Comparison Journalists (N=107)		Analysis			
	N	%	N	%		Fisher's Exact Test, Two-Sided (p)		
Cannabis use	34	24.3	20	18.7		0.29		
Use of other substances[a]	9	6.4	2	1.9		0.12		

	Mean	SD	Mean	SD	t	df	p	95% CI of Difference
Weekly units of alcohol[b]								
Men	14.7	12.3	7.6	7.1	5.0	178.9	0.0001	4.3 to 10.1
Women	10.8	9.4	3.9	3.7	3.8	37.7	0.001	3.2 to 10.7
Scores on Impact of Event Scale—Revised[c]								
Intrusion	9.2	7.1	4.3	4.4	6.5	226.6	0.0001	3.4 to 6.4
Avoidance	6.7	6.2	3.1	4.0	5.4	229.1	0.0001	2.3 to 4.9
Arousal	4.7	4.9	2.0	2.8	5.2	215.1	0.0001	1.6 to 3.6
Total	20.2	16.0	9.1	9.5	6.5	210.1	0.0001	7.7 to 14.4
Score on Beck Depression Inventory-II[d]	10.1	7.8	6.4	6.1	4.1	235.8	0.0001	1.9 to 5.4
Scores on General Health Questionnaire[e]								
Somatic	4.4	3.4	4.2	2.9	0.6	243	0.54	−0.6 to 1.1
Anxiety	5.9	4.0	4.7	3.5	2.3	243	0.02	0.2 to 2.1
Social dysfunction	7.3	3.0	6.7	2.2	1.9	243.5	0.05	−0.0 to 1.3
Depression	2.2	3.4	1.0	2.3	3.4	239.5	0.001	0.5 to 1.9
Total	19.8	10.6	16.6	7.8	2.7	243.6	0.008	0.9 to 5.5

[a] Amphetamines, cocaine, barbiturates, heroin.
[b] A unit of alcohol was defined as a regular-size bottle of beer, a glass of wine, or a shot of spirits. Fourteen units of alcohol per week for men and 9 units for women were considered the upper limits of acceptable weekly intake (15).
[c] Number of war journalists: intrusion, N=135; avoidance, N=134; arousal, N=133; total, N=127.
[d] For war journalists, N=132.
[e] Number of war journalists: somatic, N=138; anxiety, N=138; social dysfunction, N=139; depression, N=139; total, N=138.

A significant number of war correspondents, particularly women, drink excessively, with a weekly alcohol consumption well above that of their nonwar colleagues. However, heavy drinking did not necessarily translate into a diagnosis of alcohol abuse or dependence as defined by DSM-IV. The lifetime prevalence of alcohol abuse did not differ from that in the general population (20). While heavy drinking may not have rendered the majority dysfunctional with respect to their work, it does leave the individual at risk for a host of long-term medical problems (15).

Results from all self-report measures of PTSD and depression revealed higher scores in the war group. While useful as screening instruments, self-report questionnaires cannot by themselves generate psychiatric diagnoses. Furthermore, the Impact of Event Scale—Revised, Beck Depression Inventory-II, and General Health Questionnaire provided indices of current symptoms only. These two limitations do not, however, apply to a structured clinical interview, such as the SCID. The fact that only one in five war journalists could be interviewed was due solely to logistical difficulties. The 28 journalists selected at random were scattered over three continents during the course of the study, and it often took months to finally connect and complete the process. Nevertheless, the clinical interviews corroborated the finding of significant psychopathology in approximately one-quarter of the group.

Of the 28 war journalists interviewed, all had been shot at numerous times, three had been wounded (of whom one had been shot on four separate occasions), three had

had close colleagues who were killed while they were working together on assignments, two had been subject to mock executions, two had had bounties placed on their heads, one had survived a plane crash (the pilots were killed) only to be subsequently robbed by soldiers who looted the wreckage, and two had had close colleagues who committed suicide. Given these descriptive details, higher scores on the Impact of Event Scale, an index of PTSD, were not unexpected in the war group. While symptoms from all three subscales were frequently endorsed, intrusive and hyperarousal symptoms, i.e., unwanted recollections of specific events accompanied by hypervigilance and autonomic arousal, were more common than avoidance phenomena. Of note was the fact that the avoidance item "I stayed away from reminders of the trauma" was endorsed least often. Rather, the avoidance pattern incorporated such maladaptive strategies as "My feelings about it were kind of numb" and "I felt as if it hadn't happened." Thus, despite deeply troubling recollections of events witnessed, the war journalists returned constantly to the scenes of old or new traumas, a pattern of behavior sustained over many years. This could contribute to their high lifetime prevalence of PTSD, i.e., 28.6%. In addition, the fact that PTSD, in all but one case, developed after the journalists began working in war zones suggests a strong connection between the dangers confronted in war and the development of psychopathology.

It is noteworthy that the lifetime prevalence of PTSD in war journalists exceeds the 7%–13% reported for traumatized police officers (21, 22) but is equivalent to (23) or less than (24) figures for combat veterans, depending on the source cited. Such comparisons, while placing the result within a comparative frame of reference, are nevertheless misleading. Soldiers and policemen receive extensive training to deal with violence. War journalists do not. In recognition of this deficiency, innovative trauma education programs for journalists in training have begun to be offered by some universities (25).

The high PTSD figures are matched by the rates for major depression. Once again, the figures for the war group are substantially higher than those for the comparison group. With the structured interview, the lifetime prevalence of major depression in the war group was 21.4%, which exceeds the 17.1% rate reported for the general population in the United States (20). If one removes the one subject whose major depression predated work in war zones, the prevalence drops to 14.3%. However, it is important to note that the U.S. data are made up of equal numbers of male and female subjects, and the latter have a lifetime prevalence of 21.3%, almost double the approximately 12% in males. In our predominantly male study group, even after we controlled for the cases predating war exposure, the result still translates into a lifetime prevalence of major depression above that in the U.S. National Comorbidity Study (20). The high comorbidity of major depression and PTSD in this study is in keeping with figures from trauma studies of other population groups (26, 27).

With the stringent Bonferroni correction factor applied to the data, the results from the 28-item General Health Questionnaire essentially confirmed the preceding finding with respect to depression. This instrument was used previously as an index of psychological distress in trauma settings (28, 29). The higher total scores in the war journalists were driven mostly by elevated depression scores and, to a lesser extent, symptoms of anxiety and social dysfunction.

The interviews with 20% of the group revealed that war journalists are profoundly affected by their symptoms of PTSD. While we had no clear way of judging the effects of the syndrome on the quality of their work, every war journalist with PTSD spoke of considerable social difficulties, such as an inability to adjust to life back in a civil society, a reluctance to mix with friends, troubled relationships, the use of alcohol as a hypnotic, and embarrassing startle responses that led to social avoidance. With such difficulties, they fulfilled the DSM-IV criterion that specifies that the symptoms must cause "significant distress or impairment in social, occupational or other important areas of functioning."

Perhaps our most telling observation was that despite greater levels of psychopathology than in the comparison group, the war journalists were not more likely to have received help, be it pharmacotherapy or psychotherapy. The clear implication is that many war journalists are not receiving treatment for their PTSD, depression, and alcohol abuse. The reasons for this are many and varied and not the subject of the present study. However, this observation together with the fact that we have found no previous research on this topic speak to a culture of silence on the part of the news bosses and the journalists themselves.

This last point touches on an intriguing question: What motivates war journalists to return to situations of extreme peril, particularly when almost one in four have suffered from PTSD at some point in their careers? While we plan to report this separately, a few comments are called for here. The first salient observation is that, until recently, discussing psychological distress within the profession was discouraged. A prevalent view was that to be a war journalist you had to have the "right stuff." An admission of emotional distress in a macho world was feared as a sign of weakness and a career liability. Ambition, coupled with a belief that war reporting enhances a career by giving a high media profile, left journalists reluctant to speak out about their fears and insecurities. Many chose to suffer in silence. The recent death of two celebrated war journalists on assignment in Sierra Leone (mentioned earlier) was, in part, the catalyst for a reappraisal of these views. Another, lesser factor that could have contributed to repeated exposure to trauma despite adverse consequences is the psychological naiveté inherent in some members of the profession. A number of journalists interviewed were deeply unhappy, prey to symptoms of PTSD and depression, but surprisingly unaware of what afflicted them. Thus, while giving articulate voice to subjective distress, a diagnosis such as PTSD was for the most part unknown. Such naiveté is also consonant with a belief that as a profession they can go off to war and emerge psychologically unscathed. This denial may be a necessary, albeit distorted prerequisite allowing war journalists to venture repeatedly into situations of grave physical danger.

We believe that our study is the first to explore the psychological status of war correspondents. As such, the results need replicating, more so as we were able to interview only one in five journalists. While we did not find strong evidence that psychopathology in the war group predated their exposure to war, the limited number of subjects suggests this question may not be definitively answered here. However, our findings that PTSD may affect a quarter of war journalists and that they have a high lifetime prevalence of major depression deserve serious consideration. These disorders adversely affect quality of life (30) and may tend toward chronicity if left untreated (31). The data should therefore come as a wake-up call to the news organizations that all is not necessarily well with the men and women who, at considerable risk, bring us news of the world's conflicts.

Received Aug. 6, 2001; revision received Jan. 30, 2002; accepted April 18, 2002. From the Department of Psychiatry, University of Toronto and Sunnybrook and Women's College Health Sciences Centre; and the Freedom Forum European Centre, London. Address reprint requests to Dr. Feinstein, Department of Psychiatry, University of Toronto and Sunnybrook and Women's College Health Sciences Centre, 2075 Bayview Ave., Toronto, Ont., Canada M4N 3M5; ant.feinstein@utoronto.ca (e-mail).

Supported by grants to Dr. Feinstein from the Freedom Forum and the Guggenheim Foundation.

The authors thank Vin Ray and Jackie Owen (BBC), Chris Cramer (CNN), Stephen Jukes (Reuters), Dave Modrowski (Associated Press Television News), Richard Tait (ITN), Dan Halton, George Hoff and Tony Burman (Canadian Broadcast Corporation), and Tina Carr (Rory Peck Trust).

References

1. Journalists and Media Staff Killed in 2001: An IFJ Report on Media Casualties in the Field of Journalism and Newsgathering. Brussels, International Federation of Journalists, 2001

2. Faas H, Page T: Requiem: By the Photographers Who Died in Vietnam and Indochina. New York, Random House, 1997

3. Corera G: Trends in violence and intimidation against journalists: British Broadcasting Company memo. London, BBC, 2000

4. Capa R: Slightly Out of Focus. New York, Random House (Modern Library), 1999

5. Herr M: Dispatches. New York, Vintage Books, 1991

6. Loyd A: My War Gone By, I Miss It So. New York, Atlantic Monthly Press, 1999

7. Lee KA, Vaillant GE, Torrey WC, Elder GH: A 50-year prospective study of the psychological sequelae of World War II combat. Am J Psychiatry 1995; 152:516–522

8. Wolfe J, Erickson DJ, Sharkansky EJ, King DW, King LA: Course and predictors of posttraumatic stress disorder among Gulf War veterans: a prospective analysis. J Consult Clin Psychol 1999; 67:520–528

9. Sack WH, Seeley JR, Clarke GN: Does PTSD transcend cultural barriers? a study from the Khmer Adolescent Refugee Project. J Am Acad Child Adolesc Psychiatry 1997; 36:49–54

10. Michultka D, Blanchard EB, Kalous T: Responses to civilian war experiences: predictors of psychological functioning and coping. J Trauma Stress 1998; 11:571–577

11. Epstein RS, Fullerton CS, Ursano RJ: Posttraumatic stress disorder following an air disaster: a prospective study. Am J Psychiatry 1998; 155:934–938

12. Eriksson NG, Lundin T: Early traumatic stress reactions among Swedish survivors of the Estonia disaster. Br J Psychiatry 1996; 169:713–716

13. Wang X, Gao L, Shinfuku N, Zhang H, Zhao C, Shen Y: Longitudinal study of earthquake-related PTSD in a randomly selected community sample in North China. Am J Psychiatry 2000; 157: 1260–1266

14. Najarian LM, Goenjian AK, Pelcovitz D, Mandel F, Najarian B: Relocation after a disaster: posttraumatic stress disorder in Armenia after the earthquake. J Am Acad Child Adolesc Psychiatry 1996; 35:374–383

15. Bondy S, Ashley MJ, Rehm JT, Walsh G: Low risk drinking guidelines: the scientific evidence. Can J Public Health 1999; 90:272–276

16. Weiss D, Marmar CR: The Impact of Event Scale—Revised, in Assessing Psychological Trauma and PTSD: A Practitioner's Handbook. Edited by Wilson JP, Keane TM. New York, Guilford, 1996, pp 399–411

17. Steer RA, Ball R, Ranieri WF, Beck AT: Dimensions of the Beck Depression Inventory-II in clinically depressed outpatients. J Clin Psychol 1999; 55:117–128

18. Goldberg DP, Hillier VF: A scaled version of the General Health Questionnaire. Psychol Med 1979; 9:139–145

19. First MB, Spitzer RL, Gibbon M, Williams JBW: Structured Clinical Interview for DSM-IV Axis I Disorders, Patient Edition (SCID-P), version 2. New York, New York State Psychiatric Institute, Biometrics Research, 1994

20. Kessler RC, McGonagle KA, Zhao S, Nelson CB, Hughes M, Eshleman S, Wittchen H-U, Kendler KS: Lifetime and 12-month prevalence of DSM-III-R psychiatric disorders in the United States: results from the National Comorbidity Survey. Arch Gen Psychiatry 1994; 51:8–19

21. Carlier IV, Lamberts RD, Gersons BP: Risk factors for posttraumatic stress symptomatology in police officers: a prospective analysis. J Nerv Ment Dis 1997; 185:498–506

22. Robinson HM, Sigman MR, Wilson JP: Duty related stressors and PTSD in suburban police officers. Psychol Rep 1997; 81: 835–845

23. Centers for Disease Control: Health status of Vietnam veterans: psychosocial characteristics. JAMA 1988; 259:2701–2707

24. Kulka RA, Schlenger WE, Fairbank JA, Hough RL, Jordan BK, Marmar CR, Weiss DS: Trauma and the Vietnam War Generation: Report of Findings From the National Vietnam Veterans Readjustment Study. New York, Brunner/Mazel, 1990

25. Coté W, Simpson R: Covering Violence: A Guide to Ethical Reporting About Victims of Trauma. New York, Columbia University Press, 2000

26. Bleich A, Koslowsky M, Dolev A, Lerer B: Posttraumatic stress disorder and depression: an analysis of comorbidity. Br J Psychiatry 1997; 170:479–482

27. Brady KT: Posttraumatic stress disorder and comorbidity: recognizing the many faces of PTSD. J Clin Psychiatry 1997; 58(suppl 9):12–15

28. McFarlane AC, Papay P: Multiple diagnoses in posttraumatic stress disorder in the victims of a natural disaster. J Nerv Ment Dis 1992; 180:498–504

29. Turner SW, Thompson J, Rosser RM: The Kings Cross fire: psychological reactions. J Trauma Stress 1995; 8:419–427

30. Zatzick DF, Marmar CR, Weiss DS, Browner WS, Metzler TJ, Golding JM, Stewart A, Schlenger WE, Wells KB: Posttraumatic stress disorder and functioning and quality of life outcomes in a nationally representative sample of male Vietnam veterans. Am J Psychiatry 1997; 154:1690–1695

31. Hierhollzer R, Munson J, Peabody C, Rosenberg J: Clinical presentation of PTSD in World War II combat veterans. Hosp Community Psychiatry 1992; 43:816–820

Suggested Reading

American Psychiatric Association. *Diagnostic and Statistical Manual of Mental Disorders*. 4th ed. Washington: APA, 1994.

Anon. *The Love of an Unknown Soldier*. London: The Bodley Head, 1918.

Arnett, Peter. *Live from the Battlefield: From Vietnam to Baghdad: 35 Years in the World's War Zones*. New York: Simon and Schuster, 1994.

Baxter, Jenny, and Malcolm Downing. *The BBC Reports: On America, Its Allies and Enemies, and the Counterattack on Terrorism*. New York: Overlook Press, 2002.

Bell, Martin. *In Harm's Way: Reflections of a War-Zone Thug*. London: Penguin, 1996.

Bourke, Joanna. *An Intimate History of Killing: Face to Face Killing in Twentieth Century Warfare*. London: Granta Books, 1999.

Buell, Hal. *Moments: Pulitzer Prize–Winning Photographs*. New York: Black Dog and Leventhal, 2002.

Burton, Robert. *The Anatomy of Melancholy*. New York: Tudor, 1927.

Capa, Robert. *Slightly Out of Focus*. New York: Modern Library, 1999.

Carroll, Andrew. *War Letters: Extraordinary Correspondence from American Wars*. New York: Washington Square Press, 2001.

Challoner, Jack. *The Brain*. London: Channel 4 Books, 2000.

Chatwin, Bruce. *Anatomy of Restlessness: Selected Writings 1969–1989*. New York: Viking, 1996.

Coté, William, and Roger Simpson. *Covering Violence: A Guide to Ethical Reporting about Victims and Trauma*. New York: Columbia University Press, 2000.

di Giovanni, Janine. *The Quick and the Dead: Under Siege in Sarajevo*. London: Phoenix House, 1994.

Faas, Horst, and Tim Page, eds. *Requiem: By the Photographers Who Died in Vietnam and Indochina*. New York: Random House, 1997.

Feinstein, Anthony, John Owen, and Nancy Blair. "A Hazardous Profession: War, Journalists and Psychopathology." *American Journal of Psychiatry* 159 (2002): 1570–75.

Fialka, John J. *Hotel Warriors: Covering the Gulf War*. Washington, D.C.: Woodrow Wilson Center Press, 1991.

Gall, Sandy. *Don't Worry about the Money Now*. London: Hamish Hamilton, 1983.

Gellhorn, Martha. *The Face of War*. New York: Atlantic Monthly Press, 1998.

———. *Travels with Myself and Another: A Memoir*. New York: Tarcher Putnam, 2001.

Gourevitch, Philip. *We Wish to Inform You That Tomorrow We Will Be Killed with Our Families: Stories from Rwanda*. London: Picador, 2000.

Gutman, Roy. *A Witness to Genocide: The 1993 Pulitzer Prize–Winning Dispatches on the Ethnic Cleansing of Bosnia*. Dorset, U.K.: Element Books Limited, 1993.

Hedges, Chris. *War Is a Force That Gives Us Meaning*. New York: Public Affairs, 2002.

Herr, Michael. *Dispatches*. New York: Knopf, 1977.

Howard, Michael. *The Invention of Peace: Reflections on War and International Order*. New Haven, Conn.: Yale University Press, 2000.

Holmes, Richard. *Acts of War: The Behavior of Men in Battle*. New York: Free Press, 1985.

Howe, Peter. *Shooting Under Fire: The World of the War Photographer*. New York: Artisan, 2002.

Hudson, Miles, and John Stanier. *War and the Media*. Gloucestershire, U.K.: Sutton, 1997.

Kapuscinski, Ryszard. *Another Day of Life*. New York: Vintage, 2001.

———. *Imperium*. New York: Vintage, 1995.

——. *The Shadow of the Sun*. New York: Alfred A. Knopf, 2001.

Keane, Feargal. *Letter to Daniel: Despatches from the Heart*. London: BBC, 1996.

——. *Seasons of Blood: A Rwandan Journey*. London: Penguin, 1996.

Keegan, John. *War and Our World*. New York: Vintage, 1998.

Knightley, Phillip. *The First Casualty: From the Crimea to Vietnam: The War Correspondent as Hero, Propagandist, and Myth Maker*. New York: Harcourt, Brace Jovanovich, 1975.

Kogan, Deborah Copaken. *Shutterbabe: Adventures in Love and War*. New York: Villard, 2000.

Liebling, A. J., ed. *New Yorker Book of War Pieces: London 1939 to Hiroshima 1945*. New York: Schocken, 1947.

Loyd, Anthony. *My War Gone By: I Miss It So*. New York: Atlantic Monthly Press, 1999.

Marinovich, Greg, and Joao Silva. *The Bang-Bang Club: Snapshots from a Hidden War*. New York: Basic Books, 2000.

May, Antoinette. *Witness to War: A Biography of Marguerite Higgins*. New York: Beaufort Books Inc., 1983.

McCullin, Don. *Sleeping with Ghosts: A Life's Work in Photography*. New York: Aperture, 1996.

——. *Unreasonable Behaviour: An Autobiography*. New York: Alfred A. Knopf, 1992.

Micale, Mark S., and Paul Lerner. *Traumatic Pasts: History, Psychiatry, and Trauma in the Modern Age, 1870–1930*. Cambridge, U.K.: Cambridge University Press, 2001.

Miller, William Ian. *The Mystery of Courage*. Cambridge, Mass.: Harvard University Press, 2000.

Moran, Daniel. *Wars of National Liberation*. London: Cassell, 2002.

Nordstrom, Carolyn, and Antonius C. G. M. Robben, eds. *Fieldwork Under Fire: Contemporary Studies of Violence and Survival*. Berkeley: University of California Press, 1995.

Page, Tim. *Page After Page: Memoirs of a War-Torn Photographer*. New York: Atheneum, 1988.

Pearl, Daniel. *At Home in the World: Collected Writings from the* Wall Street Journal. New York: Wall Street Journal Books, 2002.

Pedelty, Mark. *War Stories: The Culture of Foreign Correspondents*. New York: Routledge, 1995.

Peterson, Scott. *Me against My Brother: At War in Somalia, Sudan and Rwanda*. New York: Routledge, 2000.

Politkovskaya, Anna. *A Dirty War: A Russian Reporter in Chechnya*. London: Harvill Press, 2001.

Roth, Mitchel P. *Historical Dictionary of War Journalism*. Westport, Conn.: Greenwood Press, 1997.

Russell, Alec. *Big Men, Little People: Encounters in Africa*. London: Pan, 2000.

Shawcross, William. *Deliver Us from Evil: Peacekeepers, Warlords, and a World of Endless Conflict*. New York: Simon and Schuster, 2000.

Shephard, Ben. *A War of Nerves: Soldiers and Psychiatrists 1914–1994*. London: Jonathan Cape, 2000.

Silber, Laura, and Allan Little. *Yugoslavia: Death of a Nation*. New York: Penguin, 1997.

Simpson, John. *A Mad World, My Masters: Tales from a Traveller's Life*. London: Pan, 2001.

———. *Strange Places, Questionable People*. London: Pan, 1998.

Smith, W. Eugene. *Let Truth Be the Prejudice: W. Eugene Smith: His Life and Photographs*. New York: Aperture, 1985.

Sorel, Nancy Caldwell. *The Women Who Wrote the War*. New York: Perennial, 2000.

Steele, Jon. *War Junkie: One Man's Addiction to the Worst Places on Earth*. London: Bantam Press, 2002.

Stewart, Ian. *Freetown Ambush: A Reporter's Year in Africa*. Toronto: Penguin, 2002.

Sudetic, Chuck. *Blood and Vengeance: One Family's Story of the War in Bosnia*. New York: Penguin, 1998.

Sweeney, Michael S. *From the Front: The Story of War*. Washington, D.C.: National Geographic, 2002.

Waugh, Evelyn. *Scoop*. New York: Back Bay Books, 1999.

Whelan, Richard. *Robert Capa: The Definitive Collection*. London: Phaidon, 2001.

Wolff, Tobias. *In Pharaoh's Army: Memories of the Lost War*. New York: Vintage, 1995.

Zuckerman, Marvin. *Behavioral Expressions and Biosocial Bases of Sensation Seeking*. Cambridge, U.K.: Cambridge University Press, 1994.

Acknowledgements

This book owes much to the journalists who made time in busy, often hectic schedules to fill out questionnaires and meet with me. Of those I interviewed all were prepared to be quoted, although some preferred anonymity. I have respected this need for confidentiality, which in the rare instance meant that I had to alter some personal identifying characteristics. I have not, however, changed the content of what any journalist had to say.

My study was funded by the Freedom Forum in those halcyon pre–September 11 days when the world seemed safe and life less fraught. John Owen was then the European Director of the Freedom Forum and ran what can be best described as a journalists' salon in a beautiful set of offices overlooking the greenery of Hyde Park. It was John who persuaded the Freedom Forum in Washington to fund my study and it was John who opened the doors to many of the news organizations. Without his enthusiasm and good offices I doubt whether a lot of hard-boiled news bosses would have entertained a visit from an unknown Canadian psychiatrist asking to explore the emotional lives of their employees. The London offices of the Freedom Forum are sadly no more. I, like many others, benefited from the rich cultural and academic milieu that John was able to create.

My thanks to the news bosses of those organizations that participated in my study: Stephen Jukes of Reuters, Dave Modrowski of Associated Press Television News, Vin Ray of the British Broadcasting Corporation, Tony Burman of the Canadian Broadcasting Corporation, and Richard Tait of Independent Television News. Chris Cramer, the president of CNN International, was at the forefront of this support. Over the years Chris has established a remarkable reputation as a champion of good, safe journalism, and his unwavering commitment to this project and others is gratefully acknowledged. Tina Carr of the Rory Peck Trust was instrumental in helping recruit freelance journalists and I thank her for this and her infectious energy.

Patrick Crean and Jim Gifford of Thomas Allen Publishers, Janice Weaver and Alison Reid, and Linda McKnight of Westwood Creative Artists helped my thoughts find a home and did so with tact, patience, and generosity.

This book has been written on weekends, evenings, and holidays. It has been written in the bedroom, the dining room, and hotel rooms on four continents. It has been written in time poached from family commitments. To my wife, Karen, and children Pippa, Saul and Clarrie, I add love to my thanks.

Index